Diagnostic Ultrasound in Small Animal practice

Paddy Mannion

BVMS, DVR, MRCVS, Diplomate ECVDI

Blackwell
Science

Editorial offices:
Blackwell Science Ltd, 9600 Garsington Road, Oxford OX4 2DQ, UK
 Tel: +44 (0) 1865 776868
Blackwell Publishing Professional, 2121 State Avenue, Ames,
Iowa 50014-8300, USA
 Tel: +1 515 292 0140
Blackwell Science Asia Pty, 550 Swanston Street, Carlton,
Victoria 3053, Australia
 Tel: +61 (0)3 8359 1011

The right of the Author to be identified as the Author of this
Work has been asserted in accordance with the Copyright,
Designs and Patents Act 1988.

First published 2006

ISBN-10: 0-632-05387-9
ISBN-13: 978-0-632-05387-2

Library of Congress Cataloging-in-Publication Data

Mannion, Paddy.
  Diagnostic ultrasound in small animal practice / Paddy Mannion.
      p. cm.
  Includes bibliographical references and index.
  ISBN-13: 978-0-632-05387-2 (pbk. : alk. paper)
  ISBN-10: 0-632-05387-9 (pbk. : alk. paper)
  1. Veterinary ultrasonography. I. Title.

  SF772.58.M36 2005
  636.089'607543–dc22   2005008357

A catalogue record for this title is available from the British Library

Set in 10/12.5pt Plantin
by Graphicraft Limited, Hong Kong

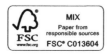

Contents

Foreword

It gives me pleasure to write the foreword to this new version of Diagnostic Ultrasound in the Dog and Cat. Diagnostic ultrasound has advanced in leaps and bounds since the book was first published in 1990. There have been major technological advances in transducer design and image acquisition and processing, resulting in images of vastly improved resolution. Despite this, the cost of equipment has come down in relative terms, and is now a viable option for many small animal practices. Owners are increasingly well informed and are often aware of ultrasound as a safe and informative diagnostic procedure. Taking all these factors into account, more veterinary surgeons than ever before are aiming to develop or update their expertise in diagnostic ultrasound.

Several authors have been involved in the writing of this new book, reflecting perhaps the expansion of the subject and the specialist expertise which an individual is now able to develop in given areas. The authors are all very well known in the field of small animal diagnostic ultrasound, and will be bringing to the reader a wealth of practical experience as well as important theoretical knowledge; both aspects are vital in acquiring the best possible images and in reaching pertinent and accurate conclusions. This book will be valuable to those who are just beginning to develop their skills with diagnostic ultrasound, as well as to those who wish to update and extend their knowledge. I am delighted to be able to recommend it to you.

Frances Barr

Contributor List

Paddy Mannion   BVMS DVR MRCVS Dip ECVDI
Cambridge Radiology Referrals
RCVS Recognised Specialist in Veterinary
Diagnostic Imaging
European Specialist in Veterinary Diagnostic Imaging

Mairi Frame   BVMS DVR MRCVS Dip ECVDI
Lecturer in Veterinary Diagnostic Imaging,
Edinburgh University Vet School
RCVS Diplomate in Veterinary Diagnostic Imaging
European Specialist in Veterinary Diagnostic Imaging

Sharon Redrobe   BSc(Hons) BVetMed CertLAS DZooMed
MRCVS
RCVS Recognised Specialist in Zoo and
Wildlife Medicine

Alison King   BVMS, MVM, DVR, DipECVDI,
MRCVS
RCVS Recognised Specialist in Veterinary
Diagnostic Imaging
European Specialist in Veterinary Diagnostic Imaging
Lecturer in Veterinary Clinical Anatomy,
Glasgow University Veterinary School

Johann Lang,
Prof   Dr.med.vet., Dip ECVDI
European Specialist in Veterinary Diagnostic Imaging
Head, Division of Clinical Radiology
Department of Clinical Veterinary Medicine
University of Bern

Valerie Schmidt   DrMedVet Cert VR Dip ECVDI
European Specialist in Veterinary Diagnostic Imaging

Chapter 1

Principles of Diagnostic Ultrasound

Paddy Mannion

Diagnostic ultrasound uses high frequency sound waves to produce an image of the body. Sound waves with a frequency greater than 20 KHz are classed as high frequency as these are outside the range of human hearing. For diagnostic purposes the frequency of the sound used is typically in the range of 2–10 MHz but as technology advances, higher frequency ultrasound is being used diagnostically and in some centres frequencies of 15 MHz and above are being used for high resolution work.

Sound waves

Sound energy is mechanical energy which means that it requires a medium for propagation as it produces physical movement of the molecules and particles within the material through which it travels. Sound waves are longitudinal waves in which the direction of travel of particles within the wave is the same as that of the wave itself. Each wave has cycles of compression and rarefaction (Figure 1.1). Each wave has an associated speed of travel, a wavelength and frequency. The wavelength is the distance travelled in one cycle, which is the distance between the same point in successive areas of compression or rarefaction. Frequency is the number of cycles per second and speed is the distance travelled in a particular time, usually one second. The relationship between these factors is shown in the following equation:

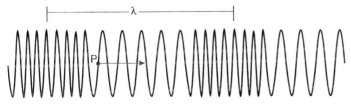

Figure 1.1 Diagram of a longitudinal wave – note the cycles of compression and rarefaction. The wavelength (λ) is shown as the distance between the centre point of successive areas of compression or rarefaction. The direction of motion of the particle (P) is the same as the direction of the wave itself.

1

$$v = f \times \lambda \quad > \quad f \, \alpha \, 1/\lambda$$

v = velocity   f = frequency λ = wavelength

1 cycle/second	=	1 Hz
1000 cycles/second	=	1 KHz
1 000 000 cycles/second	=	1 MHz

In general, the speed of travel of sound through soft tissues is taken as a fairly constant value (approximately 1540 m/s) and so wavelength and frequency are inversely related. This is fundamental to the practical application of ultrasound. Essentially, the higher the frequency of the sound waves produced, the shorter the wavelength of the sound. Examples of how this relates to commonly used frequencies are shown below.

Frequency (MHz)	Wavelength (mm)
2	0.77
5	0.31
7.5	0.21

The speed of travel of sound through different tissues varies according to their individual properties, in particular their density. Therefore, while the average speed of sound in soft tissue is 1540 m/s, through bone it is 4000 m/s and through gas it is only 300 m/s.

Material	Speed of Travel
Bone	4080 m/s
Blood	1570 m/s
Liver	1560 m/s
Fat	1440 m/s
Air	330 m/s

These differences are important as will be seen later. It is clear therefore that the transmission of sound relies on the structure of the medium and the denser the medium the faster the transmission.

Acoustic impedance

Each tissue has inherent acoustic impedance, which is essentially the resistance to the transmission of the sound wave within the material.

Acoustic impedance = Density × Speed

$$\mathbf{Z} = v \times \rho$$

Z = acoustic impedance v = velocity of sound
ρ = density of material

Acoustic impedance is important in its own right, but the difference in acoustic impedance between adjacent tissues is especially important. Where there is a great difference in acoustic impedance of adjacent tissues there is greater reflection of the sound waves from the interface of the tissues. At the interface between soft tissue and bone there is reflection of almost 50% of the ultrasound beam, whereas at the interface between soft tissue and gas this increases to almost 99%. This is very important for successful application of ultrasound as an imaging tool and interpretation of the resulting image as shown in Figures 1.2 and 1.3.

Ultrasound and tissue

The fundamental principle of diagnostic ultrasound is that sound waves pass through the tissues and are either reflected, refracted or absorbed. The sound waves which return to the transducer are responsible for producing the image. The greater the amount of sound which travels back to the transducer the brighter the image which is displayed on the screen (when using B-mode ultrasound). It is important to understand what governs the interaction between ultrasound and tissue in order to be able to interpret the image correctly. These three processes, reflection, refraction and absorption are quite different but are related.

Reflection is responsible for producing the image, as it is the reflected ultrasound waves which are transformed into the image when they reach the transducer. Reflection depends on the size of the reflecting structure and also the frequency of the sound waves in question. Higher frequency sound waves are reflected from smaller structures and are attenuated more quickly so that higher frequency sound waves are used when imaging more superficial structures. When there is a difference in acoustic impedance as the waves travel from one tissue to another there is a greater amount of reflection, as discussed above, and fewer waves remain to pass through into the deeper tissues. This explains the need for good coupling between the transducer and the skin surface.

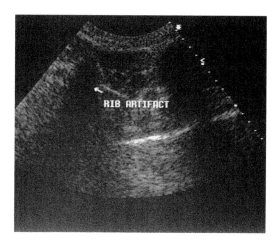

Figure 1.2 Thoracic ultrasound in a dog showing rib artefact. This image illustrates the result of 50% reflection of the ultrasound beam at the soft tissue–bone interface and absorption of the remainder of the beam within the dense bone. As a result no information is gained beyond the surface as no ultrasound passes deep to the bone. An acoustic shadow results.

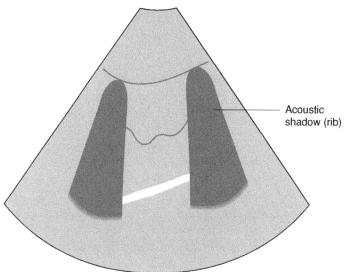

Reflection is quite straightforward when applied to the ultrasound beam, which is perpendicular to the skin surface. Where the incident ultrasound beam is not perpendicular, the reflected ultrasound beam has an angle equal to the angle of incidence, provided the speed of travel within the tissues is equal (Figure 1.4). If the speed of travel in the two tissues is different refraction occurs. Reflection from a large smooth interface with dimensions much greater than the ultrasonic wavelength, is known as specular reflection. Very often though, reflection occurs from surfaces which

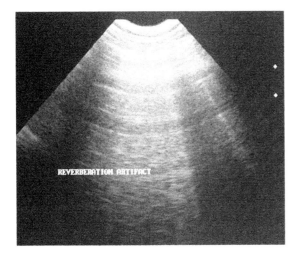

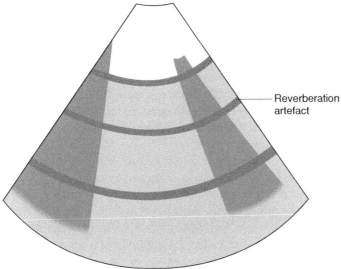

Reverberation
artefact

Figure 1.3 Thoracic ultrasound showing reverberation artefact in a dog. This image displays the effect of 99% reflection of the ultrasound beam at the soft tissue–gas interface. This poses a problem wherever there is gas.

are not completely smooth and are in the order of size of the ultrasound wavelength. These are known as diffuse reflectors as they travel in many directions and have low amplitude. This is advantageous in a way since although diffuse reflectors are weaker, they are less dependent on incident angle than specular reflectors and are used heavily to provide information on texture of the organ. Changes in scatter from one area to another are responsible for changes in brightness which are referred to as hyperechoic and hypo-echoic. A hyperechoic appearance results from an increase

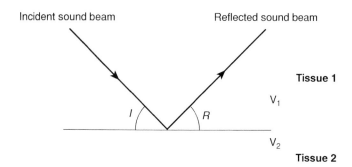

Incident sound beam   Reflected sound beam

Tissue 1

V_1

I R

V_2

Tissue 2

Figure 1.4 Where the incident ultrasound beam is not perpendicular to the interface between two structures the angle of the reflected beam (R) is equal to that of the incident beam (I), provided the speed of travel within the two tissues is the same. (V_1 = speed of sound through tissue 1, V_2 = speed of sound through tissue 2.) This is known as Snell's law.

in scattering when compared with the surrounding tissue, whereas a hypoechoic appearance results where there is a reduction in the scattering compared with the surrounding material.

Refraction is a change in direction of the sound waves as they pass from one medium into another, where the speed of travel is slightly different and occurs if the incident sound waves are oblique. Typically, this occurs where there is a fluid-filled viscus within a more solid structure, such as at the edges of the gall bladder (Figure 1.5). This is more pronounced in materials with greater acoustic impedance. As the refracted beam is travelling in a slightly different direction, the angle of reflection is also different and so the position of the imaged structure may differ from the real structure. This can produce confusing artefacts.

Where the scattering structures are much smaller than the wavelength of the incident beam and they are numerous these are known as Rayleigh scatterers. An example of this would be red blood cells. Scattering from such structures is proportional to frequency raised to the power of four so that doubling the frequency increases scattering by a factor of 16.

Attenuation is reduction in the intensity of the ultrasound beam as it passes through the tissue and occurs due to two processes; Rayleigh scatter and absorption. When sound is absorbed the energy is converted into heat by frictional forces within the tissue. This increases with the density of the material involved and explains why less sound is absorbed in fluid than soft tissue and indirectly explains the phenomenon of distant acoustic enhancement.

Attenuation is directly proportional to frequency and is also greater in tissue such as fat. This explains why higher frequency ultrasound is used at shallower depths and why

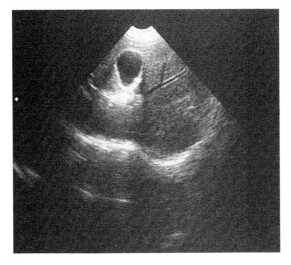

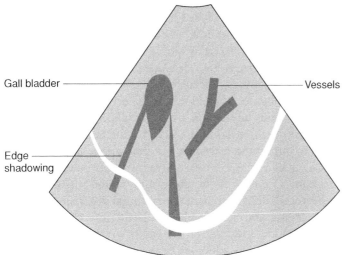

Gall bladder ——————— Vessels

Edge shadowing

Figure 1.5 This ultrasound image shows the effect of edge shadowing at the edge of the gall bladder This is caused by refraction of the ultrasound beam as the speed of travel in the fluid viscus differs from that in the liver parenchyma.

in obese animals lower frequency ultrasound may be required to obtain a diagnostic image. The following is a general guide to the depth of penetration of a particular frequency transducer:

Frequency (MHz)	Depth (cm)
5.0	12–15
7.5	6–8
10	4

Production of ultrasound

A piezoelectric crystal within the transducer produces ultrasound waves. The purpose of the transducer is twofold; to convert electrical energy into sound energy and sound energy into electrical energy in return. Typically these crystals are ceramics or composite ceramics which have been heated to very high temperatures so that they develop piezoelectric or pressure electric properties. When a voltage or potential difference is applied across the crystal it is deformed and, in response, sound waves are produced. This is known as the piezoelectric effect. The composite ceramics can now produce sound of variable frequency as chosen. The voltage is applied intermittently and the crystal will only produce sound for approximately 1% of the time. Each small package of sound is only 2–3 wavelengths. This is known as the pulse length. The transducer receives the returning echoes for the remaining 99% of the time. When the echoes are returned the crystal is deformed again and this time an electrical signal is produced which is then displayed on the screen. This is known as the inverse piezoelectric effect. The greater the potential difference applied across the crystal the greater the intensity of the ultrasound beam produced. By increasing the power the intensity of the sound beam can be increased, but it is important to remember that power and intensity are not synonymous terms. Increasing the power will increase the intensity of the ultrasound beam but increasing the power actually increases the potential difference applied to the crystal and as a result of this the reverberations are greater and the intensity of the sound produced is greater. The frequency of production of the sound waves is known as the pulse repetition frequency and depends on the length of time taken for the sound waves to return from the tissues to the transducer. Only when the echoes have been received can another pulse be submitted. When imaging superficial structures a higher pulse repetition frequency is possible and at greater depths this must be lower.

When sound is produced it is produced in all directions but only that moving in a forward motion is useful for production of an image. The transducer therefore also houses a backing block which absorbs those waves which travel backwards. It is important that the material covering the transducer does not block or reflect any of the sound waves as they pass into the tissue and therefore a special material is used.

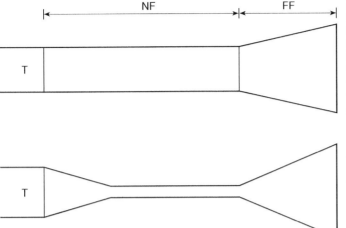

Figure 1.6a This diagram shows the shape of the unfocussed ultrasound beam as it emerges from the transducer with a narrow near field (NF) and a diverging far field (FF).

Figure 1.6b This diagram shows the effect of focussing the ultrasound beam so that there is a narrowed region of the beam where there will be improved resolution.

When the ultrasound beam is produced it diverges as it passes from the transducer into the tissues. The normal shape of the sound beam is shown simplistically in Figure 1.6, where a focussed ultrasound beam is also seen. As the ultrasound beam diverges the resolution of the ultrasound image is decreased. Resolution is an extremely important part of the ultrasound process. Spatial resolution can be divided into axial resolution and lateral resolution.

Axial resolution

Axial resolution is the ability to differentiate two points along the length of the ultrasound beam. With better axial resolution there is better image quality or detail of the image. The frequency of the transducer being used is of fundamental importance since with shorter pulse length the resolution is improved. Higher frequency ultrasound produces ultrasound with a shorter pulse length. Axial resolution cannot be any better than half the pulse length.

$$\text{Axial resolution} = \tfrac{1}{2} \times \text{Pulse length}$$

Therefore, two structures must be one pulse length apart to be recognised as separate structures (Figure 1.7).

Lateral resolution

Lateral resolution is the ability to differentiate two points lying side by side perpendicular to the ultrasound beam.

Figure 1.7   These diagrams show the principles of axial resolution. Where the two points are separated by one pulse length or more, they are displayed as separate structures on the screen. Where they are less than a pulse length apart they are seen as one point.

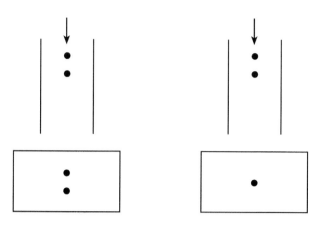

Figure 1.8   This diagram shows the principle of lateral resolution where two points perpendicular to the direction of the beam can be distinguished. Where these are within the beam they are seen as one but where they are separated by a distance greater than the beam width, they are distinguishable as separate objects.

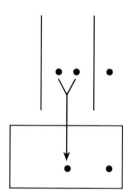

Two points which are imaged within the beam are not displayed as separate structures but two points, where one is within the beam width and the other is not, will be displayed separately (Figure 1.8). In other words if the objects are separated by a beam width they are seen as separate structures and if not they are the same structure. Higher frequency transducers have a longer near field where the beam is narrower and so have higher lateral resolution. As lateral resolution depends on beam width it is better to use a narrower or higher frequency beam or to scan in the area within the focal zone of the transducer. Most modern transducers have a focussed beam and many have a variable or even more than one focal zone where this can be adjusted to suit the image.

Ultrasound modes

A mode (amplitude mode)

Amplitude mode, or A mode, is used less often today, following improvements in real-time B-mode ultrasound. In A mode, as its name suggests, the intensity of the returning echoes is displayed on the ultrasound screen as amplitude spikes. It was used predominantly for ocular ultrasound, but specialised equipment is required which uses a single, fixed ultrasound beam and it is beyond the scope of this text to go into more detail. In some centres A-mode ultrasound is still used.

B mode (brightness mode)

B mode, or brightness mode, uses the principle that each returning echo is displayed on the screen as a dot; the brighter the dot the higher the intensity of the returning echoes. Many ultrasound beams are used and a cross-sectional image is obtained and displayed on the screen. Real-time ultrasound, where the image displayed on the screen is the image which has just been acquired and which is constantly updated, uses B-mode ultrasound (Figure 1.9). The length of time each image stays on the ultrasound screen is governed by the persistence. This may be altered on most machines. B mode, real-time ultrasound, is currently the most commonly used in diagnostic imaging.

M mode (motion mode)

M mode, or motion mode, ultrasound uses a single ultrasound beam which is in a fixed position and records how the dimensions of the section being interrogated changes with time. The image is displayed on the screen with the dimensions on the vertical or Y-axis and time on the horizontal or X-axis (Figure 1.10). This is used predominantly in echocardiography to assess dimensions of cardiac chambers and also to allow the thickness of the walls of the heart to be assessed in relation to the cardiac cycle.

The ultrasound machine

Essentially the ultrasound machine comprises the control panel with some form of monitor, either a television or

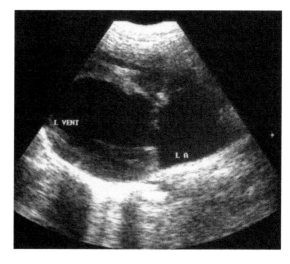

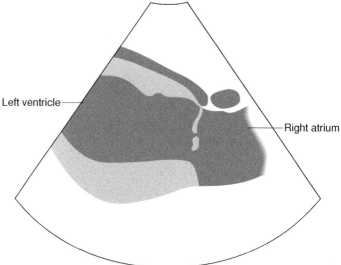

Left ventricle—

—Right atrium

Figure 1.9 A typical B-mode image of the heart. Note the left atrial dilation in this Siamese cat with cardiomyopathy.

computer screen, and the transducers. The type of ultrasound machine used governs the latter.

Control panel

The control panel of each machine will differ in layout but essentially all have similar basic controls. All have a power control, gain/reject control, TGC control, and the ability to alter both the sector angle and depth control. All allow

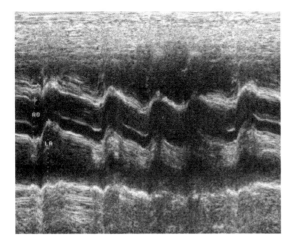

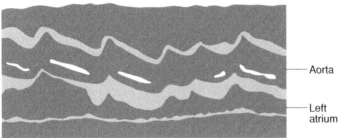

Aorta

Left atrium

Figure 1.10 A typical M-mode image showing the left atrium and the aorta.

patient identification, date and time of the examination as well as annotation of the image. Most will allow at least distance measurements.

If Doppler ultrasound is available then there are controls for choosing PW/CW (pulsed or continuous wave) or even perhaps CF (colour flow) and there may be the option to choose duplex Doppler, which is the display of a standard B-mode image and Doppler tracing concurrently. It is also possible to choose different colour maps, to zoom into areas of interest and to use a split screen on many machines.

Power

By increasing power a larger voltage or amplitude of signal is applied across the piezoelectric crystal. The effect of this is that a greater intensity of sound is produced resulting in a brighter image. An analogy which has often been used to illustrate this is that of a gong being struck; when a greater force is used to strike the gong a louder noise is produced. When a greater potential difference is applied across the crystal a greater intensity of sound is produced.

Gain/reject

Gain is the degree of amplification which must be applied to the returning echoes since these are in most cases too weak to be detected readily. The amount or degree of gain applied is the ratio of the output signal to the input signal. This is usually displayed as overall gain and time gain compensation. Overall gain is increased amplification at all levels. This should not be confused with power.

The function of the reject is to allow rejection of the weak echoes, as they perhaps do not contribute to production of a clear or good image. This should be used sparingly as some fine detail may be lost.

Time gain compensation (TGC)

This control may be in the form of twist knobs or a sliding scale. Its function is to dampen down the higher intensity echoes which return from the more superficial structures and to amplify the echoes that return from the deeper regions, resulting in a more uniform image. This control is very important for producing a high quality diagnostic image.

Persistence

This affects the length of time the image remains on the screen before it is updated. Where possible the persistence should be as low as possible to get an improved and smoother image.

Sector width

The angle of the sector image can be changed on most machines and in general for overview work the angle is quite wide, but for high resolution work it is better to use a smaller angle which will use a higher frame rate.

Frame rate

This is the rate at which the images are updated on the display. This is affected by the type of examination, such as whether cardiac or abdominal; the depth of scanning, (higher frame rates are possible at shallower depths) and the angle of interrogation (with a narrower sector width there is a higher frame rate).

Split frame

In many machines it is possible to display two or more images on the screen so that images can be compared side by side. This is not to be confused with duplex scanning where B mode and Doppler or M mode can be displayed simultaneously.

ECG

This is used in the cardiology packages so that an ECG can be displayed concurrently with the B-mode, M-mode and Doppler images. It is usually possible to switch this function on and off.

Pre- and post-processing

These controls allow manipulation of the signals both before they are stored in the scan convertor of the machine (pre-processing) and after they have been stored, but before they have been displayed (post-processing). These controls must be used with caution as it is possible to manipulate the image adversely and therefore lose valuable information. Usually they have been set by the ultrasound manufacturers but may need to be reset for each type of application such as cardiac, abdominal or vascular.

Transducer types

The ultrasound transducer or probe is a key part of the ultrasound system. Transducers are classified according to whether they are mechanical or electronic and according to the shape of the field of view they produce. In most cases the latter can be seen from the shape of the probe itself. Most transducers at this time use an array of crystals rather

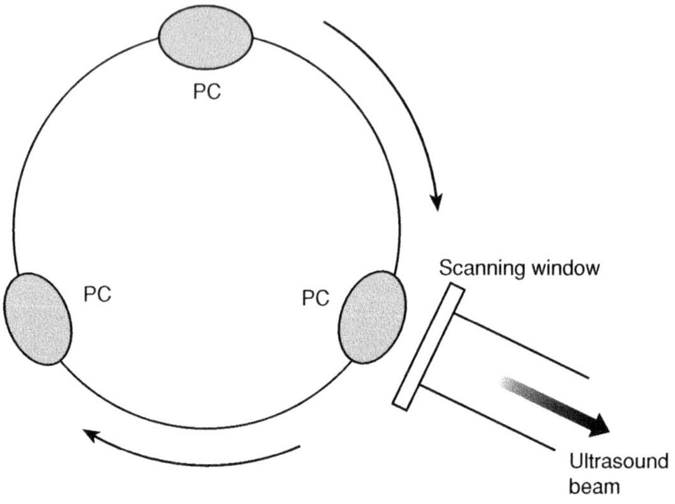

Figure 1.11 This diagram shows the basic construction of a mechanical sector transducer with the crystal elements arranged around the rotating wheel. The elements are swept past the scanning window. PC = piezo-electric crystal.

than a single crystal element. There are four main types of arrays in existence and use: linear array, curvilinear array, phased array and annular array. Only the latter is mechanical, the other three allow electronic steering. All four allow control of the beam width and focal distance.

Mechanical probes contain two to four crystals, on the rim of a rotating wheel. These are mechanically swept across the field of view to produce a fan-shaped or sector image (Figure 1.11). As mechanical probes have moving parts they produce a less sharp image and have a greater likelihood of breakdown. In some cases the crystals may be arrayed in concentric rings; these mechanical annular array transducers also produce a high quality image and may in some cases be slightly better than electronic linear arrays for detecting small focal masses. However they do not produce such good and reliable colour flow and Doppler signals as the electronic probes. Sector angle can be changed on most machines with a wider sector used to obtain an overview, while for better resolution a narrower sector is used with a faster frame rate.

Electronic probes have an array of crystals which are electronically fired to produce the image. The sequence in which this happens determines the shape of the field of view. Linear array transducers have a large number of rectangular crystal elements arranged in a line; sequential groups of these are fired intermittently to produce a rectangular image. There may be up to 250 elements with groups of up to 20 fired off each time. When the signal has returned to the transducer the next beam is fired off and this is from the parallel and adjacent group of crystals. This process is continued to the end of the array and then started over again. The whole scan takes in the order of $^1/_{30}$ of a second. This is repeated continuously and the image replaced each time on the screen. The advantage of this type of transducer is that there is a wide field of view with good definition of structures in the near field. The disadvantage is that there is a wide footprint, which restricts its application.

Curvilinear and phased array transducers produce a sector-shaped image, which is the shape of a section of a pie chart. Curvilinear arrays are really an adaptation of linear arrays and so are very similar in construction except that the crystal elements are laid out on a convex surface and the beam lines are not parallel but emerge like spokes on a wheel. These have a much bigger footprint than the phased arrays but they do have the advantage that the beam is perpendicular to the surface of the probe whereas the phased array transducers steer the beam off to the side so that it is non-perpendicular to the probe. This is to try to pick up echoes from the edges of the field but very often this is insensitive and there may be poor resolution at the edges of the image.

The phased array transducers have fewer elements, approximately 128. These transducers are smaller than the linear and curvilinear and so the elements are also narrower. All of the elements are fired off each time and beam steering is possible using time delay methods. One advantage of phased array over linear and curvilinear arrays is that there is a smaller footprint allowing access between the ribs so that these are suitable for echocardiography. The angle of the sector can be changed on most machines with the wide sector allowing a broad overview but the narrower beam providing more detail. For echocardiography a small footprint is necessary to allow access between the ribs and therefore curvilinear probes are not suitable. Phased array or microconvex probes may be suitable in these cases. The size of the footprint is the determining factor in choice of probe in veterinary practice where the small size of the patient body surface makes large probes inappropriate.

Image recording

Once the returning sound has been converted into energy at the transducer, the information is then passed to a scan convertor which stores the information and allows it to be displayed in a recognisable form such as on a TV or computer monitor. In most cases it is necessary to have some record of some or all of the examination and so it is important to be able to keep some hard copy. This may be in the form of photographic film such as in a multi-format camera, thermal printing, videotape recording or in many of the modern systems by digital archiving. For each particular system a range of options will be available and this should be discussed with the manufacturers or their representatives.

Biological safety

Biological safety of ultrasound is a complicated and as yet unresolved issue and the purpose of mentioning it in this book is to alert users to the potential complications that do exist. It is beyond the scope of this book to explore this issue fully and so the reader is directed to other texts for this (see Suggested Reading section at the end of the chapter).

It appears to be clear that ultrasound remains the safest of the diagnostic imaging modes given the potential effects of X-rays, gamma rays and even MRI. However, ultrasound can have potentially damaging effects such as tissue heating, cavitation and bruising if used irresponsibly.

The thermal effects of ultrasound are perhaps seen most at the body surface and at the surface of bone where increases in temperature of 2–3°C are quite possible. As cells may be damaged by extremes of temperature, it is important that the ultrasound mode be correctly set for mechanical and thermal indices.

Acoustic cavitation is commonly cited as a potential side-effect of ultrasound but this has not been proven where there are not pre-existing gas bodies.

Bruising is a potential problem but not usually at current diagnostic levels and any bruising would be expected to repair in a normal way.

As use of ultrasound increases it is clear that ideas on the safety of ultrasound are developing but this is still being researched. This data has been adapted from the literature in the field of human ultrasound.

Suggested reading

Boon, J. A. (1998) The Physics of Ultrasound. In: *Manual of Veterinary Echocardiography*, 1st edn, pp. 1–34. Lippincott Williams & Wilkins, Hagerstown, MD.

Curry III, T. S., Dowdey, J. E. & Murry Jr, R. C. (1990) Ultrasound. In: *Christensen's Physics of Diagnostic Radiology*, 4th edn. Leo & Febiger, Philadelphia.

Duck, F. A. (2 Jan 2003) Working Towards the Boundaries of Safety. In: *EFSUMB Newsletter*, **16**, 8–11.

Nyland, T. G. & Mattoon, J. S. (2002) Physical Principles, Instrumentation and Safety of Diagnostic Ultrasound. In: *Small Animal Diagnostic Ultrasound*, 2nd edn, pp. 1–18. W. B. Saunders Co., Philadelphia.

Zagzebski, J. A. (1996) *Essentials of Ultrasound Physics*. Mosby, St Louis.

Chapter 2

Ultrasound Artefacts

Johann Lang

Unlike radiographic artefacts, many ultrasound artefacts may be useful and a clear understanding of what they signify may be helpful with interpretation of an image. Improper use of the equipment, in particular when setting the controls, poor technique or inadequate patient preparation, may affect the quality and interpretation of an ultrasound image.

The artefacts discussed in this chapter are caused by physical interaction between the ultrasound beam and matter and are not due to improper scan technique.

Acoustic shadowing

Acoustic shadowing is produced by structures such as gas or bone, which reflect and/or absorb nearly 100% of the ultrasound beam (Figure 2.1). The result is that no echoes pass beyond the surface into the deeper tissues and this is displayed on the resultant image as a bright, echogenic line at the surface while the distant area is anechoic or black. This is known as acoustic shadowing. Both 'clean' and 'dirty' acoustic shadows have been described. Urinary

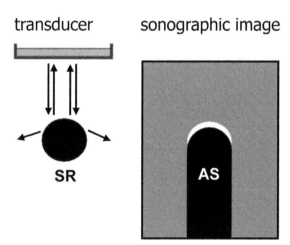

Figure 2.1 Acoustic shadowing. Structures with high attenuation (strong reflectors: SR) lead to complete reflection and/or absorption of the sound energy. Therefore, the reflective border of these structures is highly echogenic (white), while the area distant to such structures appears anechoic (acoustic shadowing: AS).

calculi (Figure 7.13, p. 135), gall stones, some foreign bodies (Figure 4.6, p. 47 distant to the suture – 'FADEN' = suture), or barium within the intestine behave in a manner similar to bone, reflecting and absorbing almost the entire sound energy and usually producing a completely black area distant to the object. This is described as a 'clean' shadow. Gas may produce a clean shadow, but can also lead to multiple reflections and reverberations thus creating an inhomogeneous or 'dirty' shadow. The type of shadow created therefore not only depends on the type of the object, but also on the size, composition and surface of the structure, as well as its position relative to the focal zone of the transducer.

A special type of acoustic shadowing, called edge shadowing, is produced at the lateral margins of cystic and other rounded fluid-filled structures such as gall bladder and urinary bladder, and may even be seen at the renal margins (Figures 2.2, 7.3, p. 117). Edge shadowing is caused by refraction of the sound beam at a fluid–tissue interface and is mainly due to different speed of sound through tissue and fluid with the rounded borders of a cyst acting as 'lens'.

Acoustic enhancement

The energy of the ultrasound beam is attenuated as it passes through tissue. While travelling through a structure with low attenuation, the sound beam loses less energy than in the surrounding tissue. The result is an increase in the strength

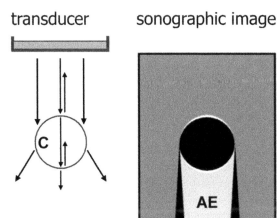

transducer   sonographic image

Figure 2.2 Edge shadowing. The lateral margins of a cyst (C) act as a lens deviating the sound beam either laterally or medially, thus creating an area with no echoes (Edge shadowing: ES) lateral to the area with acoustic enhancement (AE).

transducer   sonographic image

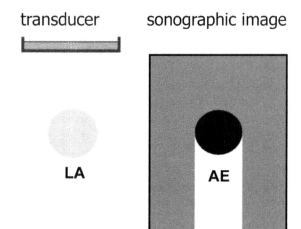

Figure 2.3 Acoustic enhancement. The area distant to structures with low attenuation (LA) presents with increased echogenicity (AE).

of echoes returning from distant to this structure and this is displayed as an area of increased brightness on the screen (Figures 2.3, 7.3, p. 117). This mainly occurs distant to fluid-filled structures such as the gall bladder, urinary bladder or any cystic structure and is helpful in differentiating hypoechoic from fluid-filled structures. However, some solid hypoechoic structures may also show some distant acoustic enhancement.

Reverberation

Reverberation artefact involves reflection of the ultrasound beam backwards and forwards between the transducer and a highly reflective surface (Figure 2.4). This occurs commonly at the interface of the transducer and the body wall (external reverberation) but can occur at the interface of any highly reflective surface in the path of the ultrasound beam such as the small intestine or between the body wall and lung (internal reverberation).

Using thoracic ultrasound as an example, the ultrasound beam passes from the transducer, through the chest wall into the tissues and is reflected back to the transducer from the surface of the lung by the air. The transducer records this returning echo and an echogenic line is shown on the image. The echo bounces back to the lung surface and is again reflected back to the transducer. This is recorded but as this echo has travelled twice the distance and has taken twice as long to come back the ultrasound machine records it as having originated deep to the first. This is repeated

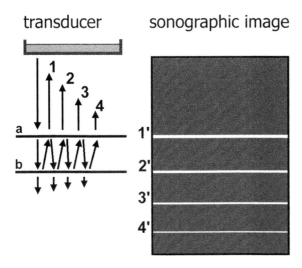

transcducer   sonographic image

Figure 2.4
Reverberation. Here the sound beam is bouncing back and forth between the two strong reflectors (a, b), creating multiple echoes from one pulse (1–4). Because they arrive at a later time at the transducer, the echoes are displayed as lines deeper in the image or distant to the reflectors (1′–4′).

numerous times and concentric lines are displayed on the image. No information is gained beyond the surface and this explains why ultrasound has limited use for investigation of pulmonary disease and also why acoustic windows are so important for echocardiography. Comet-tail artefact is a special form of reverberation artefact and is characterised by regular bright continuous echoes. This tends to be produced by small superficially located foreign bodies or gas bubbles.

Mirror-image artefact

An ultrasound image is generated by transforming the time taken by the ultrasound beam to be reflected back from the tissues to the transducer into a location or depth, assuming that the ultrasound beam travels in a straight line to and from the reflector (Figure 2.5). Strongly reflective concave and convex interfaces such as the diaphragm–lung interface will reflect the sound beam back into the adjacent organ such as liver, where the echo is reflected back to the diaphragm–lung interface, from where it eventually is reflected back to the transducer. Because this echo has taken longer to return to the machine than if it had travelled in a straight line, and the computer assumes that the path of the beam has been straight it also assumes its origin has been in front of the diaphragm. Mirror-image artefact must not be confused with a diaphragmatic rupture or hernia and it is important to note that it is not seen in the presence of pleural effusion.

Figure 2.5 Mirror-image artefact. A strong, obliquely oriented surface with high acoustic impedance (R) may reflect the sound beam into an organ. Objects (O) reflect the sound beam back to this surface and from there to the transducer. Because of the longer return time of the sound waves, the object will be misplaced distant to the reflector (VO = virtual object).

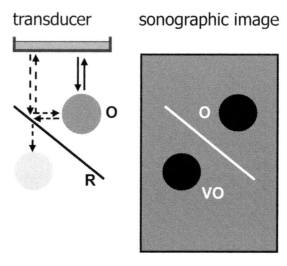

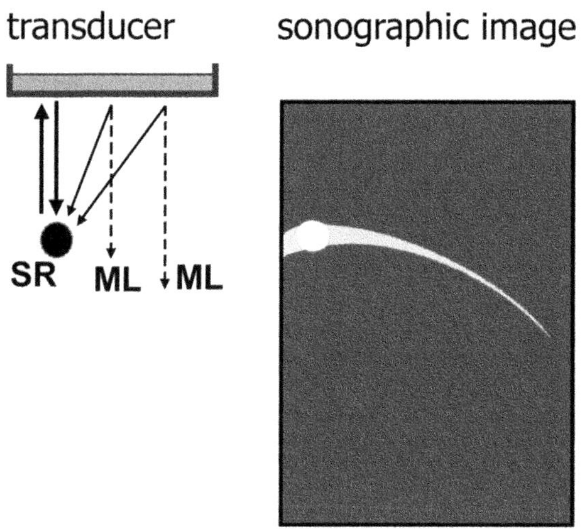

Figure 2.6 Side-lobe artefact. Strong reflectors (SR) in minor beams off the main sound beam can create echoes which are misplaced in the path of the respective main lobes (ML).

Side-lobe artefact

The ultrasound beam is composed of a main lobe and weaker secondary lobes, or side lobes. Normally, the image results from reflective objects in the path of the primary beam. However, highly reflective interfaces in the path of a side lobe can also result in an echo returning to the transducer. The returning echo will be 'misplaced' into the path of the main lobe. This artefact is generated if curved surfaces and strong reflectors such as air are present (Figure 2.6).

A variant of the side-lobe artefact is slice-thickness artefact, created in structures like the gall bladder and the urinary
bladder. It mimics the presence of sediment within these
structures and is called 'pseudo sludge' (Figure 7.10b, p. 130).
Normally, if the entire width of the sound beam is placed
within the bladder, pseudo sludge will disappear. True sediment can be differentiated from pseudo sludge by changing
the position of the patient as it remains on the dependent
side. The surface of the pseudo sludge will always be perpendicular to the sound beam.

Suggested reading

Barthez, P. Y., Leveille, R. & Scrivani, P. V. (1997) Side Lobes and
    Gating Lobe Artefacts in Ultrasound Imaging. In: *Veterinary Radiology
    and Ultrasound*, **38**, 387–393.
Curry III, T. S., Dowdey, J. E. & Murry Jr, R. C. (1990) Ultrasound. In:
    Christensen's Physics of Diagnostic Radiology, 4th edn, pp. 323–371. Leo
    & Febiger, Philadelphia.
Herring, D. S. & Bjornton, G. (1985) Physics, Facts and Artefacts of
    Diagnostic Ultrasound. *Veterinary Clinics of North America – Small
    Animal Practice*, **15**, 1107–1122.
Kirberger, R. M. (1995) Imaging Artefacts in Diagnostic Ultrasound: A
    Review. In: *Veterinary Radiology and Ultrasound*, **36**, 297–306.
Nyland, T. G. & Mattoon, J. S. (2002) Artefacts. In: *Small Animal Diagnostic
    Ultrasound*, 2nd edn, pp. 19–29. W.B. Saunders Co., Philadelphia.

Chapter 3

Indications and Technique

Paddy Mannion

Indications

Rarely should ultrasound be considered a substitute for radiography and usually it is only one of several investigative procedures to be carried out. The indications are varied and include obvious abnormalities such as a palpable mass or an audible cardiac murmur where the area of examination is clear. On some occasions the examination may be prompted by abnormal haematological or biochemical parameters and on other occasions may be as a result of clinical findings such as haematuria, jaundice or weight loss, where the underlying cause is not clear.

In most cases survey radiography must precede ultrasound and two projections of the area of interest, taken at right angles to each other, are considered as standard. Exceptions to this include respiratory distress where restraint for radiography may prove too stressful for the patient, or for pregnancy diagnosis where ionising radiations should be avoided. Where neoplasia is suspected, thoracic radiographs taken to check for pulmonary metastatic spread may also be appropriate. Usually right and left lateral projections taken on inspiration are preferable. The radiographs must be examined for abnormality and for any factors which might affect the quality and reliability of the ultrasound examination.

Patient preparation

The patient preparation required prior to the ultrasound examination is fairly straightforward. Preferably, the animal should have been starved for at least 12 hours prior to the examination. Food and gas in the stomach makes assessment of the lumen impossible and may obscure surrounding structures. In addition, faecal material in the colon may also obscure surrounding structures and precludes full

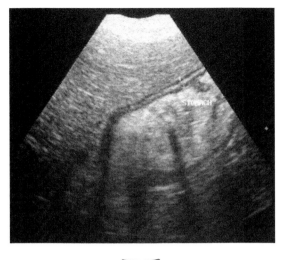

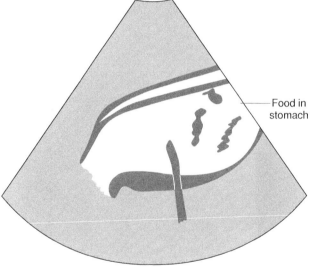

—Food in
stomach

Figure 3.1 This
ultrasound image
illustrates the effect
of the stomach full of
ingesta and gas. It is
impossible to assess
the gastric wall fully
and some of the
surrounding structures
are obscured.

assessment of the colonic wall, rendering the examination
incomplete. Unless a full bladder is helpful for the ultrasound examination, animals should be given the chance to
urinate and defecate prior to the examination. Figures 3.1
and 3.2 show the effects of a full stomach and a full colon.
In order to get good images it is essential to have good
contact between the transducer and the skin surface. This is
not possible unless the animal has been shaved or clipped,
since air trapped between the hair follicles leads to some

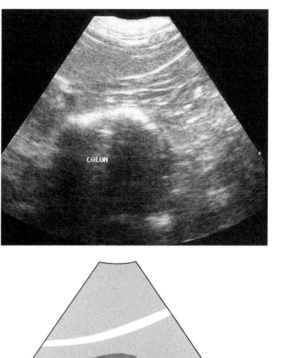

Full colon

Figure 3.2 This ultrasound image shows a full colon. The colonic wall is seen on one side only and the deeper structures are obscured.

reflection of the sound beam, reducing the quality of the image. Patients must therefore be clipped prior to the examination. This may prove a problem with some show animals but it is important to remember that the risk of missing or misinterpreting a lesion is quite great and so if clipping is not possible it is preferable not to perform the examination at all. Most clients are understanding of this if it is explained in advance. Particular recommendations for the preparation of specific areas are given in the appropriate chapters.

Patient restraint

In most cases, small animal patients are fairly compliant and will allow themselves to be positioned and held by the ultrasound helper without complaint. In some cases if the patient is comfortable they may even go to sleep during the examination. Some patients find the whole experience traumatic and in these cases some form of chemical restraint is necessary. Full details of sedative protocols are beyond the scope of this book and so general trends only are discussed. The details given here assume that the drugs used are safe given the particular situation of each patient.

For dogs there is a variety of sedative combinations available and details of these with dose rates and contraindications can be found in most current formularies. Generally for dogs a combination of acepromazine and buprenorphine has proved to be safe and effective when used appropriately. Combinations of diazepam and buprenorphine have also been used to good effect but given the effects of drugs such as α_2 agonists, agents such as medetomidine should perhaps be avoided.

For cats the various formularies provide sedative protocols with dose rates and contraindications. In clinically well patients where only mild sedation is required, a premedicant dose of acepromazine and buprenorphine combined is a good choice. When used appropriately the combination of ketamine and midazolam or diazepam is widely recognised to produce safe and effective results in patients where a greater sedative effect is required. This combination may be less effective when used in highly strung patients such as the oriental breeds and provision of a quiet and dark environment may be important for increased efficacy. In sick and older patients buprenorphine alone is often sufficient if gentle restraint only is required. In many cases a lower dose of sedation can be used or sedation dispensed with altogether when a cat muzzle is used. These are inexpensive and are invaluable in any ultrasound clinic.

Technique

There is a number of different ways in which to conduct an ultrasound examination but some standard rules apply.

Patient position

For echocardiography standard approaches are used and these are described in some detail in Chapter 10. For abdominal imaging the animal may be placed in right lateral or dorsal recumbency for the examination; which is chosen is a matter of personal preference. However, it is often the case that many examinations, if thorough, will require the patient to be placed in right-lateral and dorsal and often in left-lateral recumbency as well. The size and shape of the patient, the area of interest and the pathology present dictate this. For non-cardiac thoracic examinations the animal is usually placed with the affected side uppermost. In some situations where there is a small volume of free fluid or where the lesion is separated from the thoracic wall by a small volume of air-filled lung, it may be preferable to have the affected side dependent to reduce these effects. Therefore, the position chosen is such that the area of interest is fully and clearly seen. It can also be helpful to use positioning to reduce the deleterious effects of gas within the organs.

System

The systematic approach for echocardiography is discussed fully in the relevant chapter. For abdominal imaging the examination must be conducted in a systematic manner so that each organ is examined from left to right and from cranial to caudal in two imaging planes, sagittal and transverse. This reduces the possibility of missing small but important lesions.

The pattern in which the organs are looked at is immaterial in many ways and it is more helpful to adopt a rigid system of examination. It is often helpful to start with the liver as the hyperechoic interface between the lung and the diaphragm is such an important landmark when imaging the abdomen. The liver is examined fully in two planes and then the liver echogenicity and texture compared with that of the nearby spleen, the falciform fat and the adjacent right kidney. This provides a logical sequence in which it is automatic to look at the liver and compare it with the other organs. It is natural to scan these organs fully while looking at them and the left kidney is almost automatically scanned to compare and contrast with the right. Next, the adrenal glands may be found when in the region of the kidneys, followed by the bladder and finally the stomach and rest of the intestinal tract, including the pancreas. It is important to include an examination of the aortic bifurcation to assess possible medial iliac lymphadenopathy, which may be present in a number of conditions. For the same reason the mid-abdominal area must be checked for problems within the mesenteric nodes.

Transducer

Choosing the correct transducer is important. Usually in small dogs and cats a 7.5 or 10 MHz transducer may be used. It is often helpful with larger dogs to start the examination using a lower frequency, such as a 5 MHz transducer, and then swapping over to a higher frequency, which will allow a more detailed examination of the individual organs. This provides a general overview before looking at more specific changes. Echocardiography even in small dogs is usually best performed using a 5 MHz transducer. For areas such as the thorax, a sector, phased array or microconvex transducer is preferred, as these allow uninterrupted penetration between the ribs. For areas such as the abdomen and small parts such as the thyroid, a linear or curvilinear type, as well as the sector and microconvex varieties are suitable. In deep-chested breeds, trying to access the most cranial part of the abdomen with a linear or curvilinear probe can be difficult as they have a large footprint, or end, which will not fit easily under the ribcage; in these cases a sector transducer may be more practical. It is outside the scope of this text to provide an exhaustive list of all transducer types but in general the higher frequency will provide greater resolution but poorer depth imaging. A general guide is that 5 MHz probes will image to a depth of 15 cm adequately, 7.5 MHz will image to 7 cm and 10 MHz will only image well to a depth of 4–5 cm. These are the most commonly used frequencies in small animals, but in some very large breed dogs it may be necessary to use 2.5–3.5 MHz, especially for echocardiography. When choosing a transducer, as well as looking at frequency it is useful to look at the size of the footprint. For small parts and small animals, the smaller the footprint the better the skin contact and the easier the examination.

Further diagnostic procedures

Once the examination has been completed it is helpful to summarise the changes which have been seen and think of the differential diagnoses which may be appropriate. It is important at this point to remember that in most cases a specific diagnosis cannot be attributed to a particular sonographic picture. There are of course exceptions to this but in general a diagnosis is confirmed by a combination of the ultrasound appearance and the result of some form of biopsy procedure.

Biopsy technique

There are several biopsy techniques which may be used and which one is chosen depends on the pathology present, the organ of interest, the experience of the operator and the animal. Needle aspirate biopsy is the least invasive of all techniques. This is safe and is tolerated well by most patients, although occasionally some may react adversely, particularly where there is associated pain. With the exception of collapsed patients or where any form of sedation and analgesia is contraindicated for health reasons, and these are few, it is preferable to give the patient a combination of sedation and analgesia prior to the biopsy. In some cases it may be necessary to anaesthetise fully, particularly if the area of interest is very small and respiration must be controlled. Complications reported following ultrasound-guided biopsy include haemorrhage or haematoma at the site, local or generalised peritonitis, tumour seeding, pancreatitis, haematuria and hydronephrosis. However, there is a low rate of complications reported. Contraindications include bleeding disorders and uncontrollable patient movement.

Needle aspirate biopsy

Needle aspirate biopsies are carried out using 18–22 gauge needles. The term 'fine-needle aspirate biopsy' is reserved for needles of 20–22 gauge. Needle aspirate biopsy procedures carry very little risk of haemorrhage from the site unless it is a particularly cavitated structure such as might be found with certain tumours, as in haemangiosarcoma. These cavernous areas are best avoided in any case as often there are fewer cells contained within them and these are of reduced diagnostic quality. However, it is still a potential risk and all efforts should be made to minimise the chances of it occurring. The finest gauge needle possible is used and clients must be warned about the potential risks prior to starting. Knowledge of the animal's haematological status is important as this allows an assessment of the level of red cells and platelets. If concerned, a whole blood clotting time and buccal mucosal bleeding time can be easily and inexpensively carried out just prior to the biopsy procedure.

Fine-needle aspirate biopsy is usually carried out using a 20 gauge or smaller needle and many workers prefer the 22 gauge varieties. Special handles are available which, when placed on the syringe, create and maintain a vacuum and allow single-handed operation. It is possible to purchase needles which have been designed for tip enhancement so that the tip is more readily seen on the screen, but for the veterinary profession these are expensive, and spinal needles or hypodermic needles are generally appropriate. A good compromise for length and gauge are 22 gauge spinal needles. It is preferable to have a needle which is at least 1 inch long, and in some cases, for the deeper areas such as liver and kidney, a length of 3.5 inches may be required. In order to achieve accurate siting of these longer needles a needle guide is usually necessary, though many operators prefer a freehand technique for the more superficial structures (Figures 3.3 and 3.4). The benefit of spinal needles is that they have a metal stylet; this may be left in position until the tip is positioned within the area of interest and the stylet is then removed prior to aspiration. The clipped skin surface must be cleaned and prepared aseptically to reduce the likelihood of introducing infection into a body cavity. It is possible to get sterile sleeves for the transducer and it is

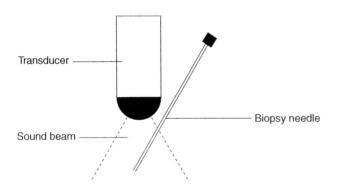

Figure 3.3 Freehand biopsy technique. The needle is introduced adjacent to the transducer, in the same plane as the sound beam.

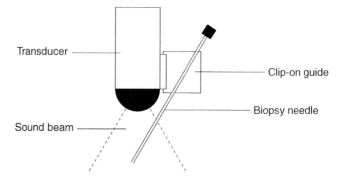

Figure 3.4 Biopsy technique using a clip-on guide. The needle is introduced through the channel in the guide.

possible to sterilise gel packs so that sterile gel is available. However, it appears that thorough cleaning of the skin and the probe and paying attention to detail ensures a safe procedure. There is still debate as to whether aspiration or suction is more beneficial. Again operator preference may influence choice but how useful the technique is may be influenced by the site of sampling, as suction is often less helpful in the spleen but is beneficial in the liver. One commonly used method does not use aspiration. The needle is introduced into the area of interest within 10 seconds and the needle moved quickly and confidently backwards and forwards up to 8–10 times before being withdrawn. The material is then blown on to a glass slide and air-dried smears made using a recognised technique. These are then submitted to a suitable laboratory. It is helpful to choose a laboratory where the cytologist is happy and confident interpreting needle-aspirate biopsy samples. The angle of the needle relative to the transducer depends on the type of transducer used and whether the entire length of the needle or the needle tip is to be shown. A skin entrance angle of 45° is appropriate for a sector transducer but a shallower angle is required for liner or curvilinear probes. Needle-aspirate biopsies may be carried out in almost any organ and it is too exhaustive a list to go through the exact procedure in each case. This technique is also extremely useful for any structure which is seen to be abnormal including lymph nodes and superficial lesions, such as body wall lesions etc.

Tissue-core biopsy

Core biopsies, as the name suggests, are biopsies where a core of tissue is removed by using a cutting cannula with a biopsy needle. These are usually half cylindrical as they have a side notch (tru cut-type samples) but it is also possible to get needles which will produce a full cylindrical sample. Most commonly 14–18 gauge automatic needles are used but occasionally 20 gauge may also be used. It is especially important to check the animal's haematological status before carrying out this type of procedure and it should include a standard haematology profile, backed up with a whole blood clotting time and, if appropriate, based on the case history, a full clotting profile.

Core biopsy needles are available in a number of different forms some of which allow single-handed operation and once primed these can be operated by pressing a button while others require two-handed operation to advance the stylet once the needle is in position. Some are available as biopsy guns where the firing mechanism is maintained within a housing and a new needle is inserted before each use, while others are a single, spring-action unit. The majority have a notched stylet, which is advanced to the area of interest and once the needle tip is in position, a cutting cannula is fired to obtain the sample. As a result these are not full cylindrical samples and have been crushed and then cut. Some newer needles are also available where a full cylindrical core is obtained. In these there is an end-cutting technique so that the sample is not crushed. The needle is introduced into the biopsy area and a set of cannulas (inner/cutting and outer/pincer) pushes forward. The inner, or cutting, cannula stops first, immediately followed by the pincer cannula, which is responsible for cutting off the sample.

Which type of core biopsy is chosen depends to some extent on the tissue type undergoing biopsy as well as on operator preference and cost, as some of the biopsy guns are very expensive. It is possible to get needles in a range of throw lengths and even some with adjustable throw lengths. Although designed for single use, in the veterinary field they are often sterilised and reused. According to a recent study, this has not been shown to have a detrimental effect on the quality of the sample obtained. The entry site is anaesthetised locally and the site of injection can be marked either by producing a skin indentation using the end of the needle cap or by using a skin marker such as marker pen. The latter often disappear during skin preparation. Aseptic skin preparation is imperative to reduce the risk of infection. The entry site is pre-cut using a number 11 scalpel blade.

The needle is introduced so that the tip is visualised, bearing in mind that if the cutting cannula throws beyond the needle tip there must be clear visualisation of the entire length of the throw. This is especially important for areas such as the liver where there are innumerable blood vessels and close proximity to the gall bladder and bile ducts. For some biopsy needles the tip is advanced proximal to the area undergoing biopsy. Each manufacturer will produce clear guidelines on the use of each particular product. In some areas, such as the kidney, it is generally felt that the needle should be rotated prior to removal as this is more likely to prevent the sample being lost.

The biopsy sample is then placed immediately in a small pot of formalin saline. It is preferable to take at least three samples, as although each sample may look adequate it is not possible to gauge their quality without laboratory analysis. The range of architecture found in the sample determines the quality and this varies between organs. In a recent study it was found that the quality of splenic core biopsies was inadequate and although there was a reasonable success rate with obtaining biopsies from the liver and kidney not all were of adequate quality.

Core biopsies are appropriate in certain regions including mediastinum, neck, liver, kidney and prostate. It should be remembered that although this is a safe procedure it does carry a risk of haemorrhage and damage to surrounding structures, with a recognised chance of obtaining an inadequate sample – in some cases it may be preferable to suggest a full surgical biopsy with a small incision technique. This type of core biopsy should not be performed on an outpatient basis and patients should remain hospitalised for 24 hours with careful observation for haemorrhage over the first 4–6 hours. If there is concern, the ultrasound scan could be repeated, looking for evidence of free abdominal fluid or the patient's packed cell volume could be checked and compared with the pre-biopsy result.

Suggested reading

Lieve, M. J. H., de Rycke, H., van Bree, J. J., *et al.* (1999) Ultrasound-guided Tissue-core Biopsy of Liver, Spleen and Kidney in Normal Dogs. In: *Veterinary Radiology and Ultrasound*, **40**:3, 294–299.

Mattoon, J. S., Auld, D. M. & Nyland, T. G. (2002) Abdominal Ultrasound Scanning Techniques. In: *Small Animal Diagnostic Ultrasound*, 2nd edn, pp. 49–81. W. B. Saunders Co., Philadelphia.

Menard, M. & Papageorges, M. (1995) Technique for Ultrasound-guided Fine Needle Biopsies. In: *Veterinary Radiology and Ultrasound*, **36**, 137–138.

Nyland, T. G., Mattoon, J. S., Herrgesell, E. J., *et al.* (2002) Ultrasound-guided Biopsy. In: *Small Animal Diagnostic Ultrasound*, 2nd edn, pp. 30–48. W. B. Saunders Co., Philadelphia.

Chapter 4

Imaging of the General Abdomen

Johann Lang

Imaging procedure

Indications for general abdominal ultrasound include disease of the abdominal organs, suspected primary or metastatic neoplasia, generalised lymphadenopathy, ascites, abdominal pain, trauma or abnormal blood results. The abdominal vessels may be imaged where there is a suspected porto-systemic shunt, tumour invasion or thrombus formation, and the large abdominal vessels often serve as land marks for other structures, such as lymph nodes or adrenal glands. The body wall and diaphragm may be assessed where there is a query regarding integrity.

In most cases, a full abdominal scan should be carried out even though a specific area is under evaluation. Where there is poor radiographic contrast, such as in animals with low body fat or ascites, an ultrasound examination should be considered the imaging method of choice. In most other cases radiography and ultrasound are considered complementary procedures.

Abdominal ultrasound may be performed with the patient in dorsal, right or left lateral recumbency and, for specific reasons, in the standing position as well. The preferred position may change with the preference of the examiner, the organ or structure in question, the amount of gas in the gastro-intestinal tract, or free fluid in the peritoneal cavity. The hair coat is clipped ventrally, but for examination of the aorta and caudal vena cava, the clipped area may have to extend laterally also. In order to allow good contact between skin and transducer, cleaning the skin with surgical spirit prior to the application of acoustic gel is recommended. Some manufacturers do not recommend this with their transducers and so this should be checked in advance. For small dogs and cats, a 7.5/10 MHz sector, linear or curved array transducer is used. For larger dogs, 5 MHz transducers are usually adequate although in some giant breed dogs 3.5 MHz may be required to allow a full examination. For assessment of the body wall, a 10 MHz linear array probe is most useful but a stand-off pad may also be required, as its position is superficial.

A thorough knowledge of cross-sectional and longitudinal anatomy of the dog and cat are important for interpretation of the ultrasound images. The examination of the abdomen should be carried out in a systematic way. The order in which this is performed may be decided by the examiner but it is imperative that the same system is used each time. Starting with the liver, all controls including the TGC (time gain compensation) are adjusted to obtain an optimal image with the same grey scale in the near and the far field. After evaluating the liver, the spleen is visualised and relative echogenicity compared. Using the spleen as a landmark or window, the left kidney is assessed for size, shape and structure and again their relative echogenicities compared. Following the aorta caudally, the regional lymph nodes followed by the urinary bladder and the genital tract (uterus/prostate) can be examined. Following the right abdominal wall, the right kidney is reached just caudal to or between the last ribs and its echogenicity is compared with that of the caudate process of the liver. From this point, the duodenum can be found ventral to the kidney, between kidney and body wall. Following the duodenum from the caudal curvature in a cranial direction, the right limb of the pancreas also can be found. The adrenal glands can be found separately or at the time of interrogation of the individual kidneys.

Sonography of the aorta or caudal vena cava is normally not difficult. Starting in the sublumbar region and imaging in a sagittal direction, they present as anechoic bands with a distinct hyperechoic border running parallel to each other in the dorsal part of the abdomen, with the vein ventral and to the right of the aorta. At the level of the kidneys the two vessels separate with the caudal vena cava running in a more ventral direction through the liver until it reaches the caval foramen in the right half of the diaphragm. In a transverse section the aorta is smaller than the caudal vena cava and is pulsatile. The caudal vena cava can be compressed easily by applying pressure with the transducer. In the caudal part of the abdomen a full bladder can serve as acoustic window for imaging aorta, aortic bifurcation and caudal vena cava. The more cranial parts are imaged either from the right or left flank of the abdomen, following the sublumbar musculature, thus avoiding overlap of intestines.

From caudal to cranial the most important arteries are the left renal, the right renal, the cranial mesenteric and the coeliac arteries. On the other hand there are no veins entering the caudal vena cava between the small phrenico-abdominal veins (just cranial to the renal veins) and the hepatic veins. The portal vein is best imaged caudal to the liver from a right ventral approach. The portal vein collects blood from the pancreas, spleen and the gastro-intestinal tract except for the anal canal. It runs ventral and slightly to the right of the caudal vena cava over the body of the pancreas and the pyloric antrum and divides at the porta hepatis into the right and left branch. Using a right lateral intercostal approach the relationship of the three large abdominal vessels can be demonstrated. Using Doppler ultrasound, especially of Doppler in abdominal vasculature, is very helpful for vessel identification, differentiating arteries and veins and assessing blood flow patterns.

Normal appearance

The normal appearance of the individual organs is covered in their respective chapters. The normal body wall consists of skin, subcutaneous fat, muscle and peritoneum appearing as more or less echogenic layers (Figure 4.1). The normal diaphragm is a very thin musculotendinous plate between the thoracic and abdominal cavities and is seen as a hyperechoic line adjacent to the cranial border of the liver. Be aware, that most of the echogenicity and the reverberation artefact distant to the liver arise from the interface with the border of the lung.

Identification of normal abdominal lymph nodes can be difficult and requires good knowledge of the various abdominal lymph centres and their respective drainage system. Normal lymph nodes may be seen in growing dogs and cats and very thin animals. Some are small and round, others elongated, thin and iso- or slightly hypoechoic structures. The different lymph nodes are imaged individually depending on their exact location. The most important are listed here.

Cranially and to the right are the hepatic lymph nodes on each side of the portal vein and the pancreaticoduodenal lymph nodes at the cranial portion of the duodenum. The large cranial mesenteric nodes (up to 6 × 2 × 0.5 cm) lie along the vascular tree of the greater omentum (Figure 4.2) and the colic lymph nodes are close to the different portions

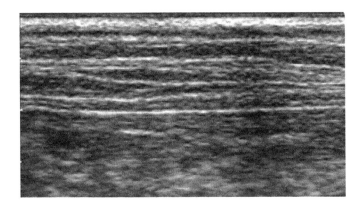

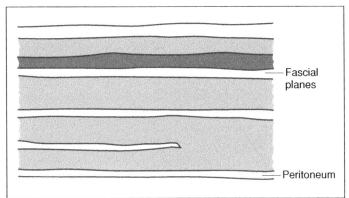

Fascial planes

Peritoneum

Figure 4.1   The normal abdominal wall consists of several layers. The hyperechoic lines represent fascial planes (arrows) while the innermost line is the peritoneum. The most superficial hyperechoic band represents subcutaneous fat and the isoechoic bands represent abdominal muscle layers.

of the gastro-intestinal tract. The splenic lymph nodes are found alongside the splenic vessels. The small lumbar lymph nodes lie alongside the aorta, the medial iliac lymph nodes between the deep circumflex and external iliac arteries and the hypogastric lymph nodes in the angle of the internal iliac and median sacral artery.

Abnormal appearance

Free abdominal fluid

Ultrasound is more sensitive than survey radiography for detecting small amounts of free fluid (4 ml/kg of body weight), especially if the animal is positioned in dorsal or sternal recumbency with the head elevated. Free abdominal fluid is seen as anechoic angular or triangular areas between abdominal structures. If a large amount of free fluid is present, the abdominal structures will be separated by large anechoic arcas, and the small intestine attached to a highly

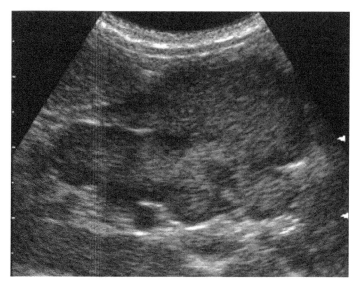

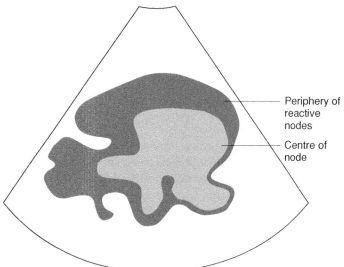

Periphery of
reactive
nodes

Centre of
node

Figure 4.2 Abdominal
scan in a dog with
chronic enteritis. The
mesenteric lymph
nodes are large and
irregular and have
smooth borders. The
centre of the node
is hyperechoic,
the periphery is
hypoechoic. Fine-
needle aspiration
revealed reactive
lymphadenitis.

echogenic mesentery is seen floating freely in the fluid (Figure 4.3). There is minimal attenuation of the ultrasound beam as it travels through fluid and the abdominal structures therefore will appear more echogenic than normal. A small effusion is best seen at the apex of the urinary bladder, delineating the serosal surface of the bladder wall or between the liver lobes, the liver and diaphragm, liver and gall bladder and also spleen and body wall. Free fluid acts as a contrast medium and is helpful for imaging abdominal structures,

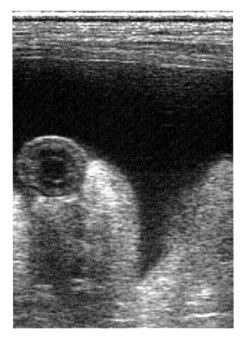

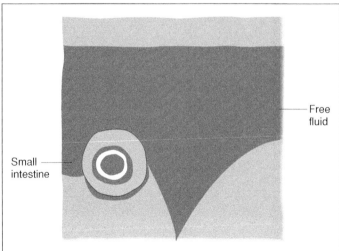

Free
fluid

Small
intestine

Figure 4.3 This dog with lymphangiectasia developed severe ascites. A large amount of free anechoic fluid is present. A transverse section of a thickened small bowel loop and hyperechoic mesenteric fat are shown.

which are sometimes difficult to visualise. Pancreas, uterus and ovaries, vessels and lymph nodes are more easily detected with free fluid in the abdominal cavity.

Retroperitoneal fluid, which may be seen where there is a ruptured kidney or ureter, accumulates around one or both kidneys, the aorta and the iliopsoas muscles. With a peritoneal effusion the fluid is normally distributed evenly throughout the abdomen. More localised fluid accumulation can be present in cases with peritonitis. Focal peritonitis associated with pancreatitis may lead to fluid accumulation in the right cranial abdomen between the duodenum, stomach, caudate lobe of the liver and right kidney. Sonographic evaluation of the fluid and the serosal surfaces can be used to characterise the type and sometimes the cause of the fluid. Completely anechoic fluid with no evidence of corpuscular echoes is typical of a transudate or modified transudate, but may be seen with a ruptured urinary bladder or gall bladder. More echogenic fluid containing multiple corpuscular echoes can be seen with haemorrhage, peritonitis, chylous effusion or carcinomatosis spread (Figure 4.4). A swirling motion may be seen within the fluid. Linear fibrinous tags within the fluid are often a sign of chronic disease. Irregular

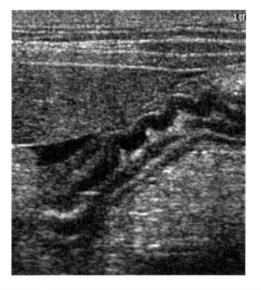

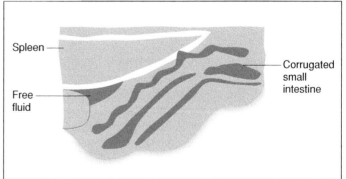

Figure 4.4 Mid-abdominal section in a dog with peritonitis. The spleen is normal. There is a small amount of free fluid adjacent to the spleen. The mesenteric fat is hyperechoic. The very irregular corrugated small bowel wall (arrows) is caused by spasticity.

serosal surfaces with increased echogenicity and stacking of intestinal structures can be a sign of carcinomatosis or chronic peritonitis (Figure 4.4).

Fluid aspiration and analysis is always necessary for diagnosis. Because free abdominal fluid is often secondary to a disease process elsewhere, it is extremely important to examine all structures and organs of the abdominal cavity and, if necessary, the thorax as well.

Intraperitoneal haemorrhage is often secondary to trauma with secondary rupture of abdominal structures, or perhaps more commonly from tumours of the abdominal viscera, especially the liver and spleen.

Protein-losing diseases, such hepatopathy, nephropathy or enteritis, portal hypertension, or increased pressure in the caudal vena cava secondary to right-sided heart failure, may all lead to the development of an abdominal effusion which is classed as a transudate or modified transudate. Intra- and retroperitoneal exudate should prompt the examiner to look for abscess formation, foreign body (Figure 4.5), pancreatitis (often localised fluid accumulation) or perforation of the gastro-intestinal tract.

Intraperitoneal urine is secondary to urinary bladder rupture. If there is retroperitoneal urine present, a ruptured kidney or ureter should be suspected.

Free abdominal air

The decubitus X-ray projection is most sensitive for detection of a small volume of free air. This requires a horizontal beam and so caution should be exercised with regard to radiation safety. Free air should be suspected if a poor quality image with reverberation artefact is seen when the patient is examined from the non-dependent side. Image quality can be improved if the patient is examined from the dependent side, but in many cases the examination must be repeated when the air has been absorbed. In some cases this may take quite some time.

Intra-abdominal masses

Abdominal masses of varying aetiology such as tumour, haematoma, cyst and abscess may originate from almost any abdominal structure. Abscesses, granulomas and haematomas have a variable sonographic appearance and may have a complex sonographic structure. A classic abscess has a thick

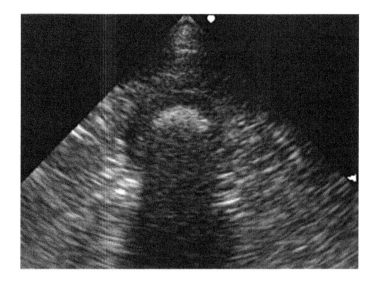

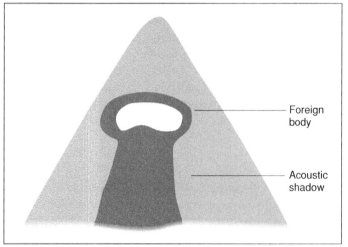

Figure 4.5 Dog with signs of peritonitis. Hyperechoic foreign body (wooden stick) with shadowing is shown in a transverse plane surrounded by a hypoechoic wall (arrows) representing reactive tissue.

Foreign body

Acoustic shadow

and irregular wall with a centre of variable echogenicity (Figure 4.6). Echogenic debris with swirling motion indicates fluid accumulation but in some cases it can be difficult to differentiate a solid hypoechoic mass from an abscess. Distant acoustic enhancement may be present. Cysts typically have a thin, well defined wall, with anechoic content, edge shadowing and distant enhancement. Tumours such as lipoma may present as homogenous hyperechoic masses or have a more mixed internal structure. Definitive diagnosis of the nature of intra-abdominal masses (neoplastic *vs.* non-neoplastic) requires ultrasound-guided biopsy or fine-needle aspiration.

Enlarged lymph nodes typically present as homogenous, hypoechoic structures with smooth borders. Sometimes

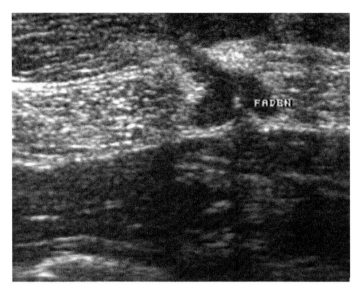

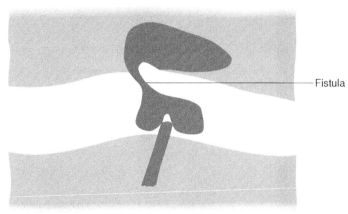

Figure 4.6 Four-year-old Boxer with a 3 year history of chronic draining fistula of the mid-ventral abdominal wall following spay. In this transverse image of the abdominal wall, an anechoic area with a hyperechoic object with shadowing is shown. This represents suture material (faden) and a fistula tract exiting at the skin near a small fluid-filled pocket.

Fistula

these may have a hyperechoic centre and are referred to as 'target lesions'. Enlarged lymph nodes may mimic fluid-filled structures if they are almost anechoic and distant enhancement may even be present. It is also possible to have a mixed, inhomogeneous appearance. In patients with lymphoma, lymph nodes of one or more centres are affected. Lymph nodes may become very large and present with irregular borders and a mixed echo pattern. Differential diagnoses for lymphadenopathy in the dog and cat include lymphoma, inflammatory disease of gastrointestinal, urogenital or pelvic structures (regional enlargement of lymph

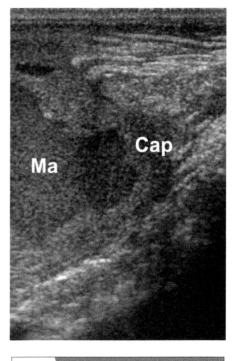

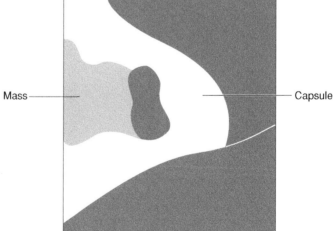

Figure 4.7 Complex mass (Ma) within the abdominal wall with a thick and irregular wall representing a capsule (Cap). The abscess contains mainly cellular material.

Mass ——————— ——————— Capsule

nodes) and metastatic spread from neoplasia elsewhere in the abdomen or pelvis.

Diaphragmatic and abdominal hernias

Ultrasound is very useful for the diagnosis of diaphragmatic rupture or peritoneo-pericardial diaphragmatic hernia, as it allows a relatively stress-free examination for the patient. This is perhaps one of the few instances where radiography is not advocated prior to the ultrasound examination. Loss of the curvilinear appearance of the diaphragm, the presence of liver or other abdominal structures close to the heart, and pleural or abdominal effusion are typical signs. An intercostal approach using a parasternal window, similar to the approach used for echocardiography, can be very helpful in establishing the diagnosis. Incomplete or small hernias may be difficult to detect. The integrity of the body wall and content of abdominal wall masses (look for bowel loops) can also be assessed (Figure 4.7). A linear transducer or a stand-off pad are helpful to evaluate superficial structures.

Suggested reading

Nyland, T. G. & Mattoon, J. S. (2002) Chapters 4 & 5: Abdominal Ultrasound Scanning Techniques; Abdominal Fluid, Lymph Nodes, Masses, Peritoneal Cavity and Great Vessel Thrombosis. In: *Small Animal Diagnostic Ultrasound*, 2nd edn, pp. 49–91. W. B. Saunders Co., Philadelphia.

Chapter 5

The Liver and Spleen

Paddy Mannion

Ultrasound of the liver

Imaging technique

Ultrasound examination of the liver is indicated when there are clinical signs or biochemical changes associated with liver disease, as well as in cases where there is vague malaise, ascites or pyrexia of unknown origin. Jaundice, weight loss, vomiting, hypersalivation and lethargy are clinical signs which might be recognised with hepatic disease.

Patient preparation is covered more fully in Chapter 3, pp. 26–29 but it is important that the patient has been starved prior to the examination, as gas and food material in the stomach may obscure certain regions, especially if the liver is small. Sedation is usually required but perhaps caution should be exercised in those patients where degradation of sedative and anaesthetic agents is compromised. In such cases, it may be preferable to use a short-acting anaesthetic agent which is not metabolised by the liver. In many cases it is possible to scan the patient without any form of restraint but for needle aspirate or other forms of biopsy, some sedation and pain relief are necessary.

The abdomen is clipped from the xiphisternum caudally but in some animals it may be necessary to clip onto the sides especially over the rib cage. This is especially important for deep-chested breeds and cases with microhepatica. The liver is scanned fully in both transverse and longitudinal sections by gently angling and moving the transducer from cranial to caudal and from right to left. Longitudinal views of the liver refer to the ultrasound beam being aligned along the long axis of the patient. The characteristic interface between the air-filled lung and the liver, which is seen as a curved hyperechoic line, is often referred to (incorrectly) as the diaphragm. The cranial aspect of the liver adjacent to the diaphragm must be examined and the caudal tips of the liver lobes also seen. The gall bladder and the porta hepatis are useful landmarks. It is often operator preference whether the patient is scanned in right lateral, left lateral or dorsal recumbency. In many cases it is preferable to use a combination of one or more of these positions, especially if the liver is small or the patient is of a less than standard body shape. The left lateral approach is often necessary where the gall bladder is of particular interest in a deep-chested patient. Some sonographers feel that hepatic examination is incomplete if the left parasternal approach has not also been used. For patients where a portosystemic shunt is suspected the standard approach is at the 11th–12th intercostal space dorsally as this ensures visualisation of aorta, then caudal vena cava and portal vein and allows inspection of a small liver.

Normal appearance

The liver has four lobes: (right/left caudate and quadrate). Blood vessels associated with the liver are the portal vein, the caudal vena cava and the hepatic veins. There is a spectrum of sonographic appearances of the normal liver ranging from a slightly coarsened appearance to a quite fine-grained tex-ture (Figure 5.1).

The normal echogenicity may vary from patient to patient. This can make assessment of diffuse disease processes very difficult and so a system whereby the appearance of the liver is compared with that of the spleen and the right kidney has been developed. This reduces the effects of normal variation and machine settings. Compared with the spleen the liver should have a reduced echogenicity and a diffuse, slightly coarse-grained texture (Figure 5.2).

Compared with the right kidney, the liver has an increased echogenicity but this relationship is highly variable as in some normal animals the liver is isoechoic compared with the kidney and in others it is hypoechoic. Therefore, while it is useful to look at both, it is felt that comparisons made between the spleen and liver are more reliable.

It is often useful to compare the echogenicity of the liver with the surrounding fat. This is especially important in cases of hepatic lipidosis in cats. The liver parenchyma is punctuated by the hepatic and portal veins, which run to the periphery of the lobes. The branches of the portal veins can be traced back to the porta hepatis where the portal

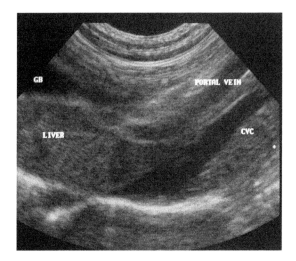

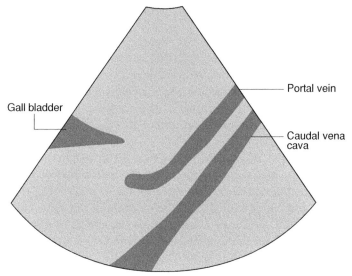

Figure 5.1   Normal liver in a cat. Note the granular texture of the normal liver. From this long-axis view of the liver highlighting the right lobes, the portal vein and caudal vena cava (CVC) can be seen.

Portal vein

Gall bladder

Caudal vena cava

vein enters. These often have echogenic walls and may be identified as vessels using either colour-flow or pulsed-wave Doppler ultrasound. If this is not available, the method of tracing them back to the portal vein as it enters the porta hepatis is usually acceptable. The hepatic veins in general have less echogenic walls and in some cases can be seen entering the caudal vena cava. This is not always the case however and again colour-flow or pulsed-wave Doppler

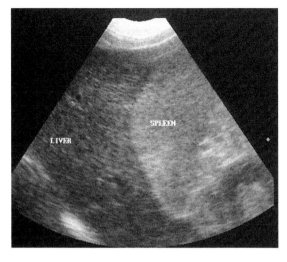

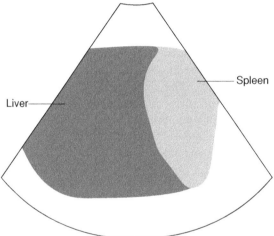

Figure 5.2 Normal liver and spleen. Note the increased echogenicity and fine-grained texture of the spleen compared to the liver – this is normal.

ultrasound may be used. The branching pattern of the hepatic and the portal veins is slightly different but the two are often seen side by side.

With the patient in lateral recumbency the gall bladder is detected as the scan is directed ventrally towards the right side. It is usually anechoic and ovoid in shape with a tapered neck. In some cats the cystic and common bile duct can be seen at the porta hepatis and this is normal if the diameter is less than or equal to 0.3 cm. It exits adjacent and slightly ventral to the portal vein. There is no flow using either pulsed-wave or colour-flow Doppler ultrasound.

The wall of the gall bladder may be seen as a very fine echogenic line and in some cases may not be very clear at all. Distant acoustic enhancement and refraction artefacts are often seen and these have been described and illustrated in Chapter 2. Although the content of the gall bladder is normally anechoic it is not unusual to get a little intraluminal sediment material. In some cases the 'sediment' is in fact due to side-lobe artefact.

As the scan is directed more ventrally the gall bladder disappears and the right lobes are picked up. As the scan is directed more dorsally the porta hepatis is imaged, and even more dorsally the left lobes are seen. The important feature of normal liver tissue is that although the texture is coarse grained it is homogeneous throughout and the caudal liver lobes have a smooth surface and are quite sharply pointed.

A thorough examination of the liver requires examination in both longitudinal and transverse planes. The ultrasound beam is aligned at right angles to the long axis of the patient and the liver is examined from right to left and cranial to caudal. This time the line of the diaphragm is seen at the bottom of the scan. The right lobes are displayed on the operator's left and the left lobes on the right. Cranially the lobes are visible as homogeneous liver tissue and more caudally the gall bladder becomes more apparent situated between the right medial and the quadrate lobes. Slightly further caudally the porta hepatis is clear with the portal vein viewed in cross section and the branches emanating from this. Slightly further caudally the right kidney is seen in contact with the caudate lobe of the liver.

Abnormal appearance

Parenchymal disease

Parenchymal disease may be typed as diffuse, focal or multifocal, and as ultrasound does not allow specific histological typing a range of differential diagnoses can exist for each appearance.

Diffuse disease

In order that the ultrasound examination of the liver can detect an abnormality suggestive of an underlying disease process there must be some disturbance of the hepatic

architecture or a change in the echotexture of the parenchyma. Where the architecture is undisturbed and only subtle
differences in texture and echogenicity exist it can be very
difficult to ascertain that this is not a normal variation.
To help in this the liver margins, the vasculature and the
biliary system are also examined. In these cases experience
of looking at many patients combined with comparison of
the liver with adjacent structures, such as the right kidney,
the spleen and the falciform fat, is very helpful. It is important that such comparisons are made at the same depth and
using the same time-gain compensation settings as changes
in these can affect the image. It is preferable therefore that
comparisons are made from the same image although it is
not always possible to do so.

The liver is usually hypoechoic when compared with the
spleen and slightly hyperechoic compared with the right
kidney. Care should be taken that the organ being compared
is not also diseased. The liver is hypoechoic compared with
the falciform fat. Differential diagnoses for diffusely increased
echogenicity in the dog must include steroid hepatopathy,
diabetic hepatopathy, hyperadrenocorticism, lymphoma
and less commonly hepatitis (Figure 5.3). Differential diagnoses in the cat must include cholangiohepatitis, diabetic
hepatopathy, hepatic lipidosis and lymphoma not in any
particular order. A diffuse decrease in echogenicity may
be seen with lymphoma, hepatitis and amyloidosis. Several
studies of cholangiohepatitis in the cat have suggested
that it is more common to see a generalised hypoechoic
appearance.

Focal disease

Where a focal lesion is found it may be helpful to try to
determine its exact location as this will help surgical planning if indicated. It is important to try to identify the extent
of involvement of the other lobes as this will help determine
if surgery is possible. In order to achieve this the liver must
be scanned thoroughly using the systematic approach. The
lobes are differentiated according to the position of the gall
bladder and the portal vein with these generally subdividing
the liver into the right and left sides. The quadrate lobe
lies ventral and to the left of the gall bladder. The caudate
lobe has a renal fossa, within which sits the right kidney,
whereas the papillary process of the caudate lobe lies just

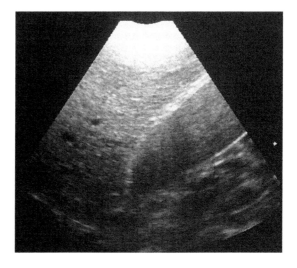

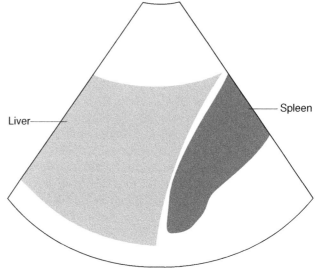

Figure 5.3 Increased echogenicity of the liver. Note the increased echogenicity of the liver compared to the spleen in this dog to whom steroids had been previously administered.

to the left of the portal vein. The left lateral lobe extends further dorsally than its medial counterpart so that it contacts the diaphragm more readily. These focal lesions may be isoechoic, hypoechoic, hyperechoic, or mixed and in some cases target lesions are seen (Figure 5.4). It is not possible to make a histological diagnosis based on the sonographic appearance and this is one of the most important principles to be understood with regard to hepatic ultrasound. Any one of the above can be found with primary neoplasia such as biliary

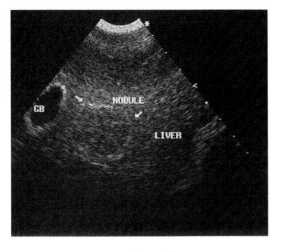

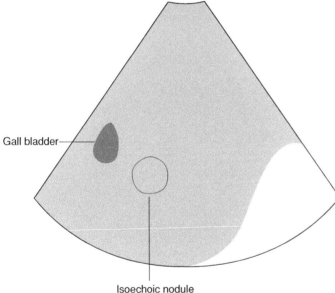

Figure 5.4 Isoechoic nodule in a dog with lymphoma. Some hepatic nodules can be difficult to delineate as can be seen in this dog with lymphoma, where an isoechoic nodule is just discernible.

carcinoma hepatoma, metastatic disease, inflammatory nodules, hyperplastic nodules and abscesses (Figure 5.5).

Target lesions are a specific type of focal lesion, which have been described in many texts. These usually have a hyperechoic or isoechoic centre and a hypoechoic rim producing a bull's eye effect. While these are associated with a strong predictive value for malignancy this is not always the case and they have been reported with benign

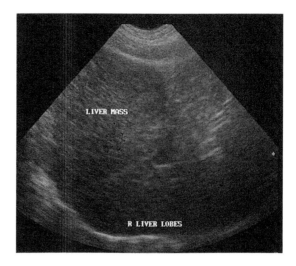

Figure 5.5 Hepatoma in a dog. An almost isoechoic mass can be seen in this 15-year-old dog with raised liver enzymes. This was diagnosed histologically as a hepatoma. In this case the mass is homogeneous but a relatively heterogeneous appearance may be seen in some cases.

hyperplasia, hepatitis and cirrhosis (Figure 5.6). For this reason identification of these lesions should be followed up with biopsy and histological typing.

Multifocal disease

This is described as a separate entity to diffuse disease as it tends to refer to more than one isolated lesion rather than an even distribution of change. There are numerous multifocal

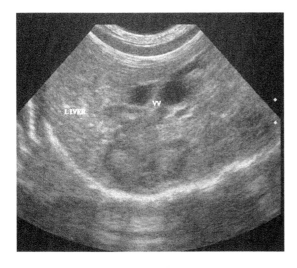

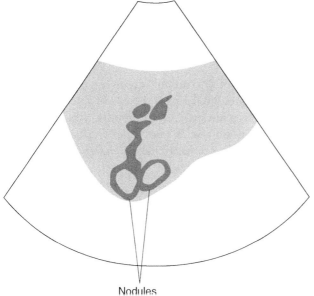

Nodules

Figure 5.6 Nodules in a cat with cholangiohepatitis. Nodules of mixed echogenicity can be seen in this cat with cholangiohepatitis. These could be described as target lesions given their ringed appearance.

diseases such as tumour metastases, benign nodular hyperplasia, cystic disease, abscesses and haematomas.

Specific conditions

Hepatic neoplasia

Liver tumours may be either primary or secondary. Primary liver tumours are considered to be uncommon and may be of epithelial or mesenchymal origin. The mesenchymal types are almost always malignant and include haemangiosarcoma, fibrosarcoma, leiomyosarcoma and extra-skeletal osteosarcoma. The epithelial tumours may in fact be benign and these include hepatocellular adenoma and cholangiocellular adenoma. The malignant epithelial forms include hepatocellular and cholangiocellular carcinomas. One form of benign condition in cats deserves particular mention – biliary cystadenomas. These are in fact the same entity as cholangiocellular adenomas. They are increasingly reported in the cat and should perhaps be considered as a differential diagnosis for any hepatic mass in an older cat. While they have a variety of presentations they usually have some cystic component. It is usually possible to differentiate these from true biliary cysts as the latter are usually very fine walled, often, though not always, solitary and contain bile when aspirated. Biliary cystadenomas are often complex and contain mucinous material rather than bile. The clinical significance of these is not clear but at this stage it is thought that they are not significant.

The liver is the most common site for metastatic spread as it filters the circulation through the portal vein (Figure 5.7). There are three main groups of tumours, which spread, to the liver: haematopoietic, in particular lymphoma; epithelial tumours such as pancreatic carcinoma; mesenchymal tumours such as haemangiosarcoma.

Benign hyperplastic nodules

These are also referred to as hepatocellular adenoma and are found in ageing dogs as a general rule. They are usually incidental findings and are not thought to be precancerous in their form. It is important that they be differentiated from metastatic nodules and biopsy is required as a wide variety of size, shape and appearance is possible.

Hepatic cysts

Hepatic cysts are found in both dogs and cats and may be an incidental finding. In some cases they may be significant where there are many cysts destroying the hepatic parenchyma or where they exist as part of the polycystic renal

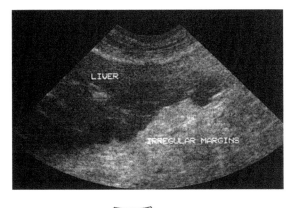

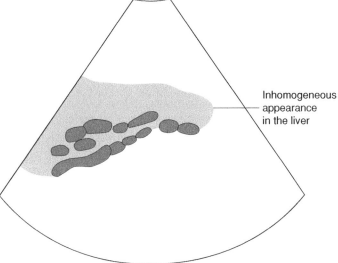

Inhomogeneous appearance in the liver

Figure 5.7   Metastatic liver disease in a dog. Note the diffuse hypoechoic nodules which can be seen in this dog with metastatic spread from an adrenal gland tumour. The liver edges are rounded and irregular.

disease complex. In general, cysts are anechoic with a fine echogenic wall and in most cases smooth margins. As with any fluid-filled structure there is generally distant acoustic enhancement and edge shadowing due to refractive artefact. In others the cysts are irregular in outline and may have irregular walls or some internal echoes and in these cases other differentials must be considered as these may represent part of another disease process such as neoplasia. It is important also to assess the rest of the abdomen, as this may be part of a polycystic problem with renal, pancreatic and hepatic involvement.

Hepatic abscess

Hepatic abscesses are not considered common in the dog and cat and a variety of sonographic appearances may be found. Most have been described as being round or oval and may be irregular in outline. They may be solitary or multiple and the content ranges from anechoic to echogenic. Differences in echogenicity can be seen within different areas of the same lesion. Some display an echogenic rim which can have a variety of thickness. Target lesions have also been described and the appearance of these has no specific marking effect as the centre may be hypoechoic and the rim echogenic and vice versa. These lesions may also be seen with neoplasia and hyperplasia. In some cases there may be an associated abdominal effusion or regional lymphadenopathy. Definitive diagnosis relies on aspiration and blood samples. Care should be taken to avoid contamination of the abdominal cavity and so perhaps this should only be attempted in small–moderate lesions, which lie deep within the parenchyma, ensuring that all material is drained. Avoid the transcostal approach in case of thoracic contamination. Larger abscesses should be addressed surgically. Culture of the content is advised.

Vascular system

The hepatic vessels include the portal vein and its branches, the intrahepatic portion of the caudal vena cava and the hepatic veins and arteries. Vascular changes may be seen secondary to other conditions such as pericardial effusion where there is portal hypertension secondary to cardiac tamponade. This is quite easily detected as the caudal vena cava and the hepatic veins have become dilated. Other conditions not uncommonly seen in animals are portosystemic shunts, which may be primary or acquired. These may be intra- or extrahepatic in origin and both may be detected using ultrasound. Confirmation of a portosystemic shunt involves a meticulous examination of the caudal vena cava and the portal vein and assessment of how these relate to each other as well as what the flow characteristics of each are. Use of pulsed-wave Doppler ultrasound is necessary to detect the abnormal flow patterns and to locate the site of the abnormal vessel. Colour-flow Doppler is very helpful in most cases as it allows the site of turbulent blood flow to be detected easily and then a more detailed examination can begin. It is beyond the scope of this book to consider colour-flow Doppler ultrasound in detail.

Biliary disease

Gall bladder

The appearance of the normal gall bladder has been described earlier in this chapter (see p. 53). The normal cystic/common bile duct can be seen in most patients. The intraparenchymal ducts are not usually seen unless dilated and they can then be differentiated from the hepatic vessels by their branching pattern and tortuous appearance. In some cases of long standing cholangitis or cholangiohepatitis the wall of the gall bladder may be quite hyperechoic or even thickened (Figure 5.8).

Obstructive disease

Obstruction of the biliary tract may occur due to obstruction of the major hepatic ducts, the cystic duct or the common bile duct. This may be due to a mural, intraluminal or extramural causes. Cholelithiasis is perhaps the most common cause of intraluminal obstruction and these are seen within the gall bladder or the bile duct as hyperechoic structures casting a strong acoustic shadow. If they are sitting within the bile duct this may be dilated and tortuous (Figure 5.9).

Mural causes of obstruction are usually due to severe inflammation or occasionally neoplasia such as bile duct carcinoma. In these cases the wall of the gall bladder may be thickened and irregular and the bile duct may appear occluded. The bile duct carcinomas may be seen as an echogenic mass within the dilated and obstructed ducts. This can also be seen where there is chronic inflammation.

Extramural obstruction can occur secondary to inflammation, infection and neoplasia of the pancreas, duodenum and cranial abdominal lymph nodes and these structures must all be assessed where there are signs of obstruction.

Mucinous hypertrophy

In many dogs in particular, the internal margins of the gall bladder often appear irregular and small nodules can be

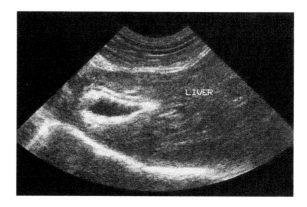

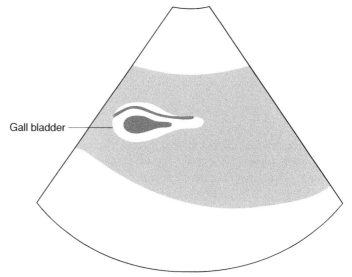

Gall bladder

Figure 5.8 Chronic cholangitis in a cat. In this cat with chronic cholangitis the gall bladder wall is thickened and hyperechoic.

seen projecting into the lumen of the gall bladder. These are usually hypertrophied mucus-producing glands and are usually an incidental finding of no real clinical significance.

Sediment

In many cases where the patient has had a variable appetite, or been inappetant for any length of time, there may be echogenic sediment within the gall bladder. It should be remembered that side-lobe artefact gives the false impression that there is sediment present. In other cases the sediment may appear quite hyperechoic and almost 'formed'

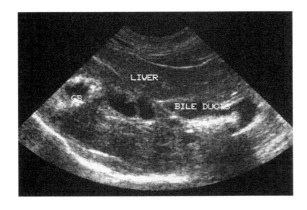

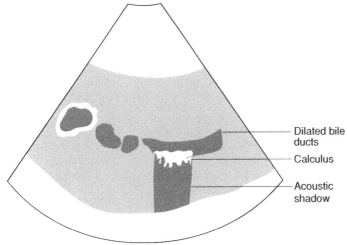

Dilated bile
ducts

Calculus

Acoustic
shadow

Figure 5.9
Cholelithiasis in a cat.
There is an obvious
partial obstruction of
the bile duct within
which hyperechoic
calculi can be seen.
An acoustic shadow is
seen distant to the
calculi.

although there is no evidence of mineralisation (Figure 5.10). This is often incidental though occasionally may be more pathological and may be associated with chronic infection.

Microhepatica

Liver size is more difficult to assess from an ultrasound examination than from a radiograph. However it is clear, where there appears to be reduced liver volume and where there is little space between the liver and intestine, that the liver size is small. In many of these patients the liver has to be examined from an intercostal approach. In these cases

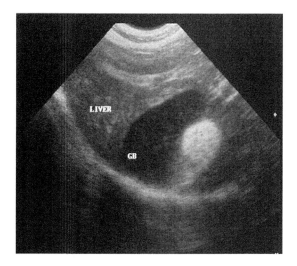

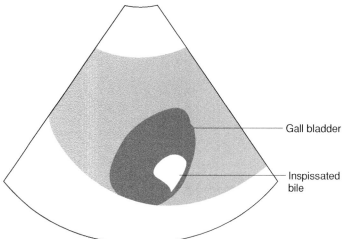

Figure 5.10
Inspissated bile in
a dog. There is
echogenic material
in the gall bladder of
this dog. The material
appears almost
'formed' although no
acoustic shadowing is
seen suggesting that it
is not mineralised.

Gall bladder

Inspissated
bile

it is imperative that they have been starved prior to the
examination as gas within the stomach can make assessment almost impossible. The two most common differential
diagnoses for microhepatica are cirrhosis and a portosystemic
shunt. Where there is a portosystemic shunt, the liver is
small and is usually poorly vascularised. The abnormal
shunting vessel may be seen relatively easily within the liver
between the portal vein and caudal vena cava or less easily
outside the liver between the renal vein and the hepatic
veins. The liver parenchyma is usually of normal to slightly
increased echogenicity and there are smooth, sharp edges

throughout the liver lobes. This contrasts with the appearance of the cirrhotic liver. In some cases there may be cirrhotic nodules present, which are isoechoic and are not easily identified. In these cases, the liver appears relatively normal. In most cases there are variably sized nodules which are mildly hypoechoic ranging through to hyperechoic. The liver margins are often rounded and irregular (Figure 5.11). In some advanced cases, where there is ongoing inflammation/fibrosis, dystrophic mineralisation may be present, seen on

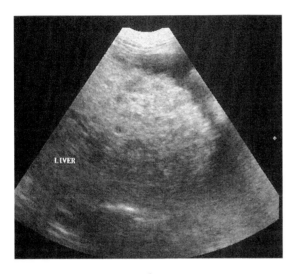

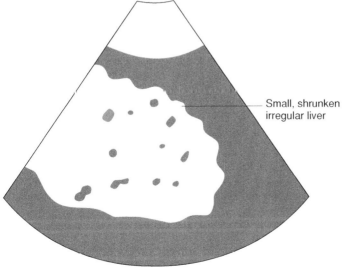

Small, shrunken irregular liver

Figure 5.11 Diffuse necrosis and cirrhosis in a dog. The liver in this geriatric Jack Russell terrier is diffusely nodular with an overall increased echogenicity and within this, hypoechoic nodules can be seen.

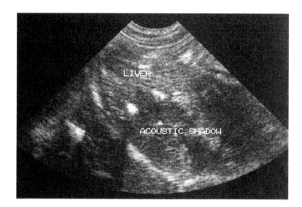

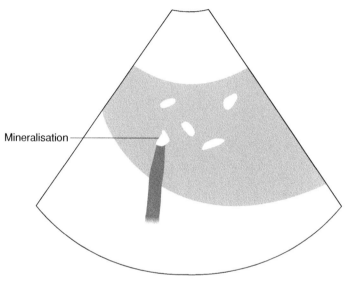

Figure 5.12 Chronic inflammatory disease in a dog. In this dog with long-term liver disease the liver is small and poorly defined. Areas of mineralisation within the parenchyma can be seen reflecting chronic inflammation.

Mineralisation

the scan as hyperechoic areas casting an acoustic shadow (Figure 5.12).

Hepatomegaly

As above, mild hepatomegaly may be difficult to detect sonographically but where it is more marked other structures are displaced and the liver can be imaged in a more caudal location. The differential diagnoses must include diabetes mellitus, hyperadrenocorticism and hepatitis. The hepatic echotexture usually has a fine-grained echogenic appearance, while, with hepatitis, this may be hyper- or hypoechoic. Needle-aspirate biopsies are usually beneficial in these cases, but a wedge or core biopsy may be required.

Ultrasound of the spleen

Imaging technique

Ultrasound examination of the spleen is indicated in instances where there is obvious splenomegaly, either radiographically or clinically, but care should be taken if the animal has been sedated with drugs such as acepromazine or has been anaesthetised using barbiturates. Other indications include unexplained anaemia, collapsing episodes or abdominal distension with fluid. In most cases the spleen is included in a general abdominal scan.

The spleen is examined with the patient in either right-lateral or dorsal recumbency. Preparation is as for the general abdomen but it is important to remember that in some cases, especially if the spleen is enlarged, the area of examination is quite large and so sufficient area should be clipped. In some cases this may extend from the xiphisternum to the groin. As the spleen is superficial avoid excessive pressure on the transducer as this may result in it not being readily seen. In most cases (including large dogs) a 7.5 MHz transducer is more than adequate to image this well and in some instances a stand-off pad may be helpful.

Normal appearance

The spleen is a straplike organ which originates on the left side of the body close to the left kidney, gastric fundus and colon. Its extent is variable depending on the degree of enlargement. The spleen has a fine-grained texture and should be wholly homogeneous (Figure 5.13). The splenic capsule is seen as a very fine hyperechoic rim and the splenic vessels are seen entering through this. In most cases, the only vessels seen are those which enter at the splenic hilus but in some cases it is possible to see many vessels entering along the length of the spleen (Figure 5.14). These can be followed for a variable but usually short depth into the splenic parenchyma. In some cases hyperechoic areas are seen around the point of entry of the vessels and these are thought to be fat deposits and nothing sinister.

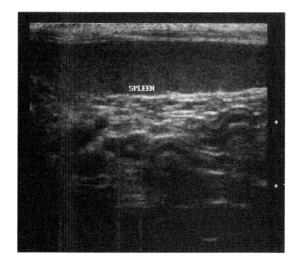

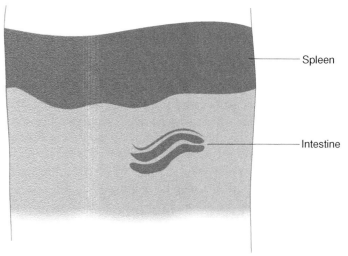

Figure 5.13 Normal spleen in a cat. The normal spleen in the cat can be seen easily with a high frequency probe. Note the strap-like appearance.

Spleen

Intestine

Abnormal appearance

Parenchymal

Diffuse

Conditions which result in diffuse splenic change include lymphoma and mast cell neoplasia (especially in cats) where there is diffuse infiltration of the organ by neoplastic cells (Figure 5.15). The spleen may appear normal in texture and echogenicity or may appear uniformly abnormal. Where there is a very uniform increase or decrease in echogenicity

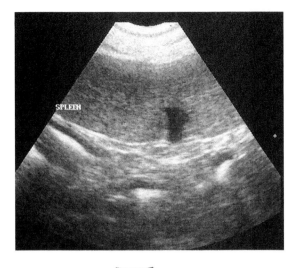

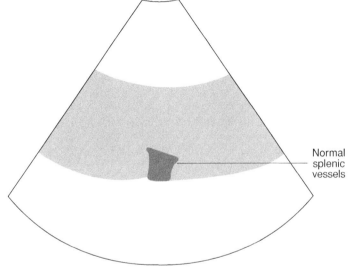

Normal splenic vessels

Figure 5.14 Normal splenic vessels in a dog. The splenic vessels can be seen entering the hilus in this case but are not traced any further into the spleen.

this can be hard to detect and it is especially important to compare this to the liver and kidneys taking care to ensure that this is done using the same TGC (time gain compensation) settings and at the same depth (Figure 5.16).

Focal

As elsewhere, focal lesions of the spleen may be hypoechoic, hyperechoic, anechoic or mixed and may vary in their size

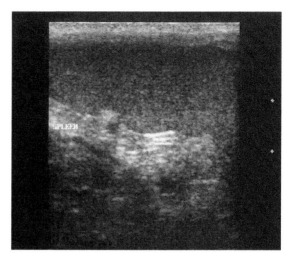

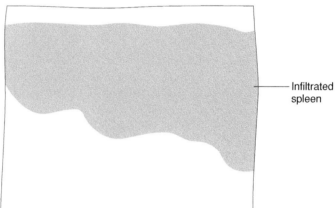

Infiltrated
spleen

Figure 5.15 Mast cell infiltrate in a cat. The spleen in this cat with diffuse spread of mast cell neoplasia is enlarged and irregular. It is perhaps slightly less echogenic than might be considered normal.

(Figure 5.17). Target lesions of the spleen have been associated with both benign and malignant conditions such as lymphoid hyperplasia, adenocarcinoma, lymphoma and haemangiosarcoma. Where there are splenic nodules it is important to realise that these are not specific for any disease process and it may be necessary to back this up with a biopsy and blood samples.

Multifocal

Many of the disease processes that affect the spleen may produce multifocal lesions and these, as above, may have a

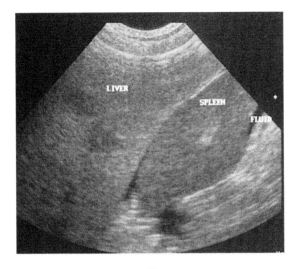

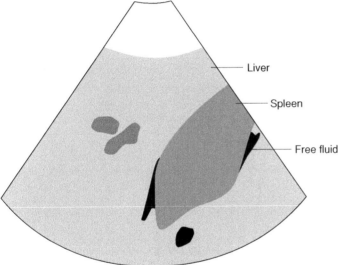

— Liver

— Spleen

— Free fluid

Figure 5.16
Reversed relationship
between liver and
spleen in a dog. The
spleen in this dog with
lymphoma has a
reduced echogenicity
compared to the liver.

range of appearances. Again, biopsy is required for definitive diagnosis.

Specific conditions

Splenic neoplasia

Splenic tumours are most frequently haemangiosarcoma/haemangioma but other masses which may present include fibrosarcoma, leiomyosarcoma, leiomyoma and lymphoma.

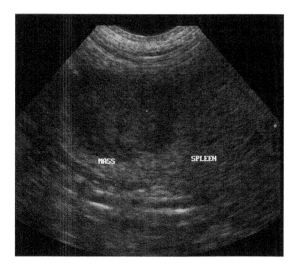

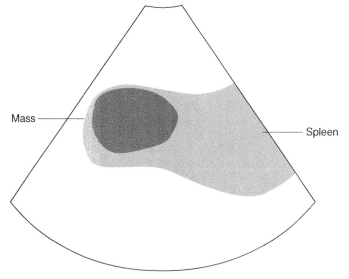

Figure 5.17 Focal splenic metastasis. A single, solid nodule can be seen in the cranial region of the spleen. This was diagnosed as a metastasis from an apocrine cell tumour.

Their ultrasound appearance is often complex with cavitated areas within which there are areas of moderate and increased echogenicity (Figure 5.18 a & b). In some cases the area of the tumour is quite small and may be surrounded by an area of haemorrhage. This can make the accuracy of biopsy quite difficult. It is important that a whole abdominal scan is performed in case of metastatic spread elsewhere and also that in some cases, especially where there is suspected haemangiosarcoma, that the heart base also be assessed.

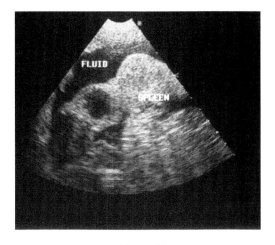

(a)

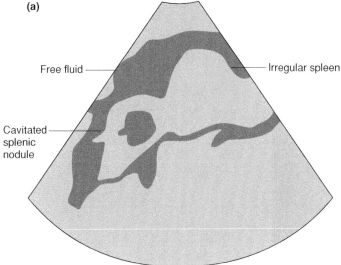

Free fluid

Irregular spleen

Cavitated
splenic
nodule

Figure 5.18a
Splenic neoplasia in a
dog. (a) The spleen
has an irregular outline
and an anechoic
nodule can be seen.
The splenic outline
is more clearly
demarcated by the
surrounding free fluid.

Splenic abscess

Splenic abscesses are not especially common in the dog
and cat but are occasionally seen. The classical presentation
is of a thick-walled, irregular structure, which may be quite
complex in echogenicity. There may be some anechoic
areas present but the fluid is usually quite echogenic due to
its cellular content. In some cases there may be gas present
and this will cast an acoustic shadow. It is impossible
in most cases to differentiate an abscess from neoplasia or
haematoma.

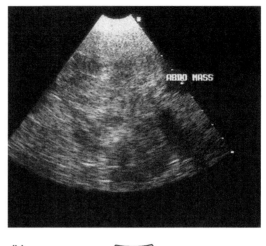

(b)

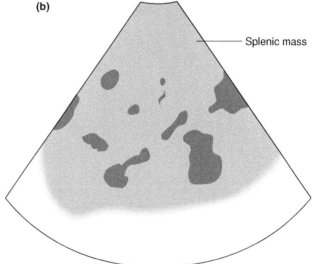

Splenic mass

Figure 5.18b
(b) A large complex mass can be seen protruding from the spleen caudally. This appearance is very typical of that seen with tumours such as haemangiosarcoma.

Splenic haematoma

Splenic haematomas may arise secondary to trauma or bleeding disorders and may present as a single or multiple masses with mainly hypoechoic and anechoic regions within (Figure 5.19). They are often complex and this may alter with age. It is important to ensure that this is an accurate diagnosis as in many cases where there are splenic tumours a haematoma may develop around the tumour.

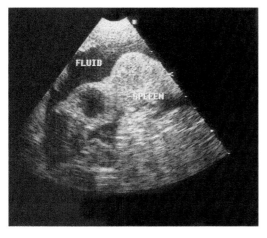

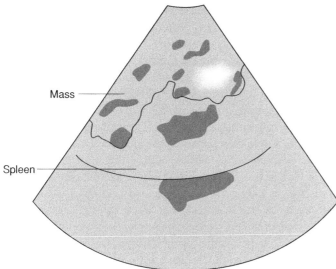

Mass

Spleen

Figure 5.19 Splenic haematoma in a dog. A large complex mass is seen in the spleen of this Bull Mastiff. This was diagnosed as a haematoma following splenectomy. It is important to ensure that there is no underlying neoplasia in these cases.

Splenic torsion

Torsion of the spleen is an uncommon condition, which may be found in association with gastric dilation-volvulus or may be found as an unrelated condition. A wide range of appearances has been described and splenic torsion should be considered as a differential diagnosis for splenomegaly. In some cases there are sonographic features of splenic congestion with dilated splenic veins and intraluminal echogenic material suggestive of vascular stasis. The splenic parenchyma may be mottled with hypoechoic areas, separated by irregular anechoic areas, suggestive of areas of necrosis, or it may be diffusely hypoechoic. In some cases the splenic parenchyma may appear homogeneous. Pulsed-wave and colour-flow Doppler ultrasound may be helpful in assessing blood flow. Almost all cases show some degree of splenomegaly.

Guided biopsy

Biopsy procedure has been described in Chapter 3, see pp. 32–36, together with indications and techniques.

In most cases it is generally agreed that needle-aspirate biopsy examination of the liver has a limited but useful application. Advantages of the technique are that it is a fairly non-invasive procedure and as such, has limited side effects, though inadvertent puncture of a blood vessel or the gall bladder are always possible. The risk of haemorrhage is quite low but this can be minimised by checking whole blood clotting time and buccal mucosal bleeding time in advance. This is particularly helpful if the procedure is carried out on an outpatient basis. Disadvantages of the needle-biopsy technique are the fact that with such a small sample the area of interest may be missed. In some conditions, such as fibrosis, the liver will not shed cells well, and so this type of biopsy is unable to type and assess the severity of the problem. Care should also perhaps be taken in these cases as the liver may not have enough elasticity to return to normal and haemorrhage may be more likely (Figure 5.20). Guided needle aspirate biopsy of the gall bladder has been described and is used when there is felt to be a need to obtain a sample for culture and sensitivity. This is a procedure that carries the risk of spillage of material (bile) into the peritoneal cavity and should be carried out with caution. Needle aspirate biopsies are felt to have benefit in detection of malignant lymphoma, hepatic lipidosis and suppurative hepatitis. Hepatocellular adenomas, hyperplastic nodules, fibrosis, chronic inflammation and neoplasia may be more difficult to detect by this method and excisional or core biopsies may be required.

Core or tru-cut biopsies perhaps have a greater value as a form of liver biopsy and should in theory produce a better sample than needle-biopsy techniques for characterisation of underlying histology. This procedure carries a greater risk than needle biopsy and as such it is important to establish

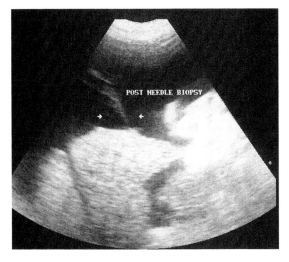

POST NEEDLE BIOPSY

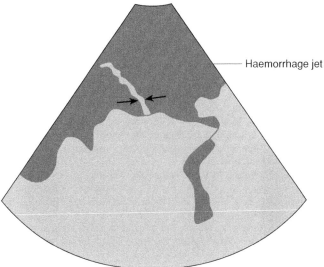

Haemorrhage jet

Figure 5.20
The large complex splenic mass was diagnosed as a haematona following spleneotomy. It is important to rule out underlying neoplasia in these cases.

clotting times in advance. It is in many cases the author's opinion that a surgical biopsy carried out through a small incision carries a lesser risk of continued haemorrhage and may also provide a more reliable sample. Sample size with core biopsy may still not be sufficient to allow hepatic architecture to be evaluated fully. Needle aspirate biopsy of the spleen has limited application. It is very useful in some cases where there may be diffuse infiltration or in cases where there are quite solid masses. In conditions where there is a cavitated appearance it is less useful, as very bloody preparations are difficult for the cytologist to interpret and may in fact not allow any further characterisation of the process which is present.

Suggested reading

Christopher, M. M. (January 2003) Cytology of the Spleen. In: *Cytology Part II. Veterinary Clinics of North America – Small Animal Practice*, **33**:1, pp. 135–152.

Cuccovillo, A. & Lamb, C. (2002) Cellular features of Sonographic Target Lesions of the Liver and Spleen in 21 Dogs and a Cat. In: *Veterinary Radiology and Ultrasound*, **43**:3, pp. 275–278.

Lieve, M. J. H., de Rycke, Henri, J. J. van Bree & Simoens, Paul, J. M. (1999). Ultrasound-Guided Tissue-Core Biopsy of Liver, Spleen and Kidney in Normal Dogs. In: *Veterinary Radiology and Ultrasound*, **40**:3, pp. 294–299.

Nyland, T. G., Mattoon, J. S., Herrgesell, E. J., *et al.* (2002) Liver. In: *Small Animal Diagnostic Ultrasound*, 2nd edn, pp. 93–127. W. B. Saunders Co., Philadelphia.

Nyland, T. G., Mattoon, J. S., Herrgesell, E. J., *et al.* (2002) Spleen. In: *Small Animal Diagnostic Ultrasound*, 2nd edn, pp. 128–143. W. B. Saunders Co., Philadelphia.

Nyland, T. G., Koblik, P. D. & Tellyer, S. E. (1999) Ultrasonographic Evaluation of Biliary Cystadenomas in Cats. In: *Veterinary Radiology and Ultrasound*, **40**:3, 300–306.

Saunders, M. H., Neath, P. J. & Brockman, D. J. (1998) B-Mode and Doppler Ultrasound Imaging of the Spleen with Canine Splenic Torsion: A Retrospective Evaluation. In: *Veterinary Radiology and Ultrasound*, **39**:4, pp. 349–353.

Schwarz, L. A., Penninck, D. G. & Leveille-Webster, C. (1998) Hepatic Abscesses in 13 Dogs: A Review of the Ultrasonographic Findings, Clinical Data and Therapeutic Options. In: *Veterinary Radiology and Ultrasound*, **39**:4, pp. 357–365.

Weiss, D. J. & Moritz, A. (November 2002) Liver Cytology. In: *Cytology Part I. Veterinary Clinics of North America – Small Animal Practice*, **32**:6, pp. 1267–1291.

Chapter 6

Gastro-intestinal Tract including Pancreas

Mairi Frame

Imaging procedure

Ultrasonography and survey radiography are the techniques most commonly used for imaging the gastro-intestinal tract. It is important to remember that these provide complementary information and are not mutually exclusive. Survey abdominal radiographs should be taken prior to a sonographic examination to assess for possible diagnosis, to rule out obvious obstruction or radio-opaque foreign body and to avoid artefact arising from residual ultrasound gel on the skin. If a barium study is required, this should be delayed until after the sonographic examination as barium degrades image quality and the enema will introduce substantial amounts of gas into the gastro-intestinal tract. However, with an experienced sonographer and suitable equipment, gastro-intestinal contrast studies become unnecessary in the majority of patients.

The advantages of ultrasound over radiography for imaging the gastro-intestinal tract are that it is a non-invasive procedure which does not use ionising radiation. The entire thickness of the bowel wall can be imaged and measured and the surrounding structures such as lymph nodes also examined. Intestinal motility can be assessed in real time and fine-needle aspirate or other forms of guided percutaneous biopsy can be performed.

Ultrasound will in most cases provide more information than a contrast study in a shorter time and with no risk of aspiration. Patient preparation is as described for general abdominal sonography (see p. 38), however the patient must be starved for at least 12–24 hours prior to examination of the gastro-intestinal tract. Standard approaches are used but advantage may be taken of fluid in dependent portions to enhance visualisation of certain structures. Ideally the gastro-intestinal tract should be examined at the end of a systematic sonographic examination of all the abdominal organs. This allows time for optimal probe contact to be achieved and for the gas in the stomach and intestines to rise to the loops of bowel in the uppermost side of the animal.

Artefact produced by gas normally found in the bowel lumen results in incomplete visualisation of the wall of the gastro-intestinal tract – a factor that should be taken into account when aiming to rule out a gastro-intestinal lesion. Various scanning techniques have been suggested to minimise the effects of gas artefact. These include imaging from the ventral aspect of the abdomen through a keyhole in the table, altering patient position or exerting mild pressure with the probe on the abdominal wall to massage gas into an adjacent section of intestine. Alternatively, the gastro-intestinal tract may be scanned obliquely from the dependent side with the patient in lateral recumbency. Scanning from both sides in this manner increases the chances of lesion detection, as does the use of at least two scanning planes for each section of the gastro-intestinal tract imaged.

Ultrasonography of the stomach wall can be misleading. Scanning obliquely can give the impression of increased wall thickness, underlining the necessity to scan in more than one plane. Measurements of wall thickness should be interpreted with caution when the stomach is empty, since the normal rugal folds can produce the appearance of gastric wall thickening or even mimic a mass. The echogenicity of the stomach wall may appear heterogeneous due to artefact arising from intraluminal gas or ingesta or through interference of ultrasound transmission by near field structures. In unclear cases, the ultrasound examination should be repeated under optimal conditions to confirm the findings, prior to any invasive procedure being carried out.

The fundus and body of the stomach lie on the left side of the abdomen immediately caudal to the liver. The pylorus lies to the right of midline in the dog and near midline in the cat. The duodenum is the only part of the small intestine which can be identified, due to its characteristic location and demonstrable connection to the pylorus. The duodenum runs from the pylorus laterally for a short distance in the right cranial abdomen, then caudally before forming a U-shaped loop at its caudal flexure. The loops of the jejunum and ileum between the duodenal flexure and the iliocaecocolic junction cannot be differentiated from one another sonographically, due to lack of reference points and the mobility of the small intestine within the abdomen. The ileocolic junction can sometimes be visualised in the right cranial abdomen as a small diameter section of intestine entering a larger diameter bowel loop; this appearance must not be mistaken for intussusception. The caecum is comma-shaped in the cat and spiral in the dog. It may be imaged in the right mid-abdominal region. The ascending colon can be traced as it runs medial to the duodenum. The transverse colon lies caudal to the stomach and left limb of the pancreas, while the descending colon runs ventral to the left kidney and dorsal or lateral to the bladder. In contrast to humans, the colon is not markedly wider than the small intestine in animals. Luminal gas hinders successful imaging of the colon and in combination with faeces can produce pseudomasses. The terminal colon and rectum, which lie within the pelvis, are largely hidden from the ultrasound beam, however the rectal wall can be examined from the lumen with a transrectal probe, if available.

Normal appearance

The wall of the gastro-intestinal tract is composed of five sonographically discernible layers, which are alternately hyper- and hypoechoic (Figure 6.1). Depending on the resolution of the equipment used and luminal content, especially gas, it may or may not be possible to recognise all five layers. Since the hypoechoic muscularis and mucosal layers pre-dominate, the overall appearance of the gastrointestinal wall is of a hypoechoic structure. The greater echogenicity of the submucosa and serosa is due to the greater quantity of fibrous connective tissue in these layers. The mucosal layer of the duodenal wall is more prominent than that of jejunum or ileum. When the layered appearance of the large intest-inal wall can be recognised, the mucosa is thinner than the other layers, which is in contrast to the situation in the small intestine. The duodenal papilla may be visible as a small hyperechoic indentation in the dorsal wall. The duo-denal wall is often slightly thicker than that in the rest of the small intestine. Small intestinal peristaltic contractions occur one to three times per minute, while peristalsis is not usually observed in the colon.

The following is a guide for intestinal thickness in dogs:

Jejunum and ileum: <20 kg – 4.2 mm >20 kg – 4.7 mm
Duodenum: <20 kg – 4.7 mm >20 kg – 5.5 mm

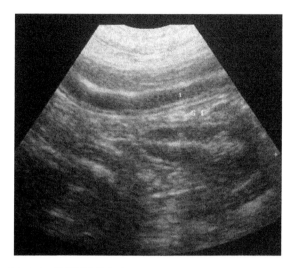

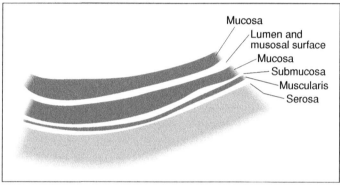

Figure 6.1 Layers of the gastro-intestinal wall.
Hyperechoic–mucosal surface and lumen.
Hypoechoic–mucosa.
Hyperechoic–submucosa.
Hypo-echoic–muscularis.
Hyperechoic–subserosa/serosa.

Mucosa
Lumen and musosal surface
Mucosa
Submucosa
Muscularis
Serosa

For the cat:

Jejunum and ileum   2.1 +/– 0.4 mm
Duodenum   2.4 +/– 0.5 mm

Normal gastric wall thickness is 3–4 mm. The normal appearance of the gastric wall is shown in Figure 6.2. Peristaltic activity is normally noted four or five times a minute in the stomach, although this may be as infrequent as once per minute if the stomach is empty.

Abnormal appearance

Inflammatory lesions of the gastro-intestinal tract

When assessing the gastro-intestinal tract for evidence of abnormality, the following features should be assessed:

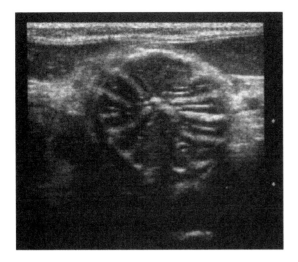

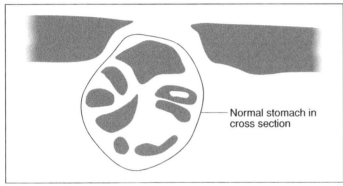

Normal stomach in cross section

Figure 6.2 Normal appearance of the stomach in a cat. Note the cartwheel appearance which is often seen when the stomach is empty.

1 wall thickness
2 wall layering
3 presence or absence of lymphadenopathy
4 involvement of other organs
5 involvement or changes in the surrounding mesenteric tissue.

The sonographic changes associated with inflammatory conditions of the gastro-intestinal tract include an increase in wall thickness or altered wall echogenicity, usually with preservation of the layering pattern and symmetry of the gastro-intestinal wall. This contrasts with neoplastic lesions, which are often asymmetrical and lead to loss of wall layering. Unfortunately, changes in neoplastic and inflammatory diseases are not specific enough to allow definitive diagnosis based on sonography alone. For example, symmetrical thickening of the wall with maintenance of the layered appearance is common with intestinal lymphosarcoma, while wall layering may be lost in fungal granulomatous conditions or severe necrosis. A few reports of muscular hypertrophy in the intestine also exist and in these the layered appearance was also lost. A wall thickness of 7 mm or more is considered abnormal in the stomach or duodenum, values of 5 mm in the dog and 3 mm in the cat are considered abnormal for the small intestinal wall.

Stomach

Sonographic findings which may be identified in gastritis include focal or diffuse thickening of the gastric wall. Gastric ulceration may also be present and in severe cases the changes may mimic a mass. Characteristic 'ulcer craters' may be difficult to demonstrate sonographically, but focal hyperechoic zones of increased gas accumulation at the mucosal surface and a spastic wall are suggestive findings (Figure 6.3). Blood clots accumulating at the site of ulceration may also appear hyperechoic. Ultrasonography can be useful to monitor complications of gastric ulceration including haemorrhage, perforation and outflow obstruction. Differentiation of benign gastric ulceration from gastric neoplasia on the basis of sonographic characteristics is not reliable since focal wall thickening with loss of layering and local lymphadenopathy may be seen in both conditions.

Sonographic findings consistent with uraemic gastropathy include thickening of the gastric wall and of the rugal folds with loss of the normal layered appearance of the wall and mineralisation of the gastric mucosa. Mucosal mineralisation appears sonographically as a highly echogenic line at the level of the gastric mucosa which produces minimal acoustic shadowing. The differential diagnosis of gastric wall mineralisation includes gastric neoplasia and disease processes causing dystrophic calcification such as primary hyperparathyroidism, hypercalcaemia of malignancy, or hyperadrenocorticism.

Chronic hypertrophic pyloric gastropathy is a condition which may be congenital or acquired and is seen especially in small breed dogs such as the Lhaso Apso or Shih Tsu. Ultrasound findings include gastric distension with fluid, gas or a mixture of these, vigorous antegrade and retrograde peristalsis failing to propel ingesta into the duodenum and

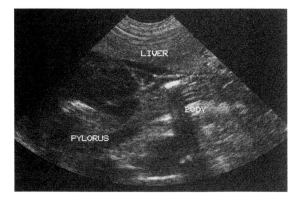

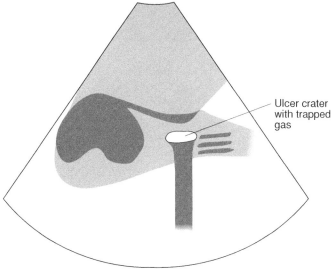

Ulcer crater
with trapped
gas

Figure 6.3 Ulcer crater. Typically a deep ulcer is seen as a hyperechoic region in the wall. This reflects gas trapped in the ulcer crater.

an even increase in thickness of the muscular layer in the pyloric canal. Gastric wall thickness is usually in excess of 9 mm with the thickness of the muscularis layer exceeding 4 mm. Diagnosis is based on the endoscopic and surgical findings and surgical biopsy.

Small intestine

Inflammatory conditions of the small intestine often produce no detectable changes in the wall, being characterised instead by atypical intestinal content and/or disturbed peristalsis. Mesenteric lymphadenopathy is frequently present.

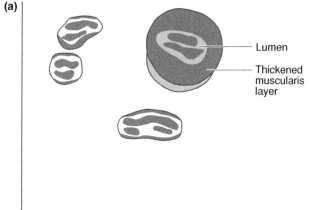

Figure 6.4 a & b
Inflammatory bowel disease. In some cases of inflammatory bowel disease the intestinal layers are present but altered and the wall is thickened. This is seen in this cat with severe, chronic inflammatory bowel disease in cross section (a) and in longitudinal section (b). The longitudinal section is also slightly dilated. In some cases the wall may be thickened though otherwise architecturally normal.

(a)

Lumen

Thickened muscularis layer

Parvoviral enteritis can cause generalised functional ileus with distended loops of small intestine lacking normal peristalsis. Inflammatory bowel disease (IBD) such as lymphocytic-plasmocytic enteritis has been reported to produce mild intestinal wall thickening with altered mucosal echogenicity and loss of layering (Figure 6.4 a & b). The intestinal loops may show a lack of definition and clarity. Ultrasound can be useful to identify abnormal sections of intestine for surgical biopsy which are not accessible endoscopically.

In the cat, it can be difficult to differentiate IBD from alimentary lymphosarcoma sonographically. Some cats with

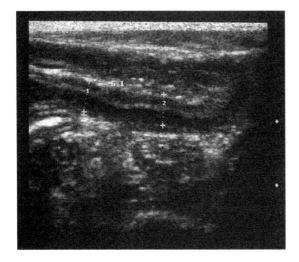

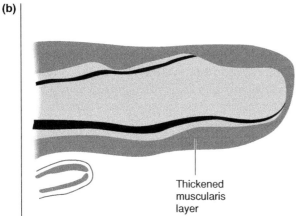

(b)

Thickened
muscularis
layer

Figure 6.4 a & b
(*continued*)

IBD will have enlarged mesenteric lymph nodes, while cats with lymphosarcoma may or may not show mesenteric lymph node enlargement. Cats with IBD may have problems involving other organ systems. A link has been made between feline IBD and suppurative cholangitis/cholangiohepatitis. The colloquialism 'Triaditis' refers to a proposed connection between IBD, hepatitis and pancreatitis in the cat.

Large intestine

Imaging of the large intestine is hindered by luminal gas and faeces, which can produce artefacts which may mask sonographic changes or mimic a mass. Diffuse thickening of the colonic wall is a non-specific change which can be due to inflammatory/infectious disease such as lymphocytic-plasmacytic colitis. Focal areas of wall thickening or mural masses may be neoplastic, polypoid or granulomatous.

Neoplastic conditions

Gastric neoplasia

Gastric neoplasia is uncommon, but occurs most frequently in middle-aged to elderly, medium to large breed dogs and in older cats. The most likely sonographic findings are a marked increase in stomach wall thickness (usually greater than 1 cm) in combination with loss of wall layering and often regional lymphadenopathy. Gastric tumours are mainly found in the pyloric antrum and may be hypoechoic, hyperechoic or of mixed echogenicity.

Carcinoma is the most common gastric neoplasm in the dog. Other gastric tumours, in decreasing order of likelihood, are leiomyoma, leiomyosarcoma, lymphosarcoma and fibrosarcoma. Gastric carcinomas have a tendency to extend beyond the serosal surface of the stomach. Leiomyomas are the most common benign gastrointestinal tumours, and are often seen as an incidental finding in old dogs at post mortem. Findings supportive of gastric leiomyoma or leiomyosarcoma are a focal mass involving the antrum with thickening of the muscularis layer of the gastric wall (Figure 6.5). Lymphoma is the most common gastrointestinal neoplasm in the cat and lesions tend to be hypoechoic (Figure 6.6).

As already mentioned, gastric wall thickening is not specific for neoplasia but may be caused by inflammatory processes. Disruption or loss of gastric wall layering is more commonly seen with neoplastic processes than with inflammatory disease. Regional lymphadenopathy may be seen in almost all conditions.

Since the identification and histological typing of gastrointestinal tumours on the basis of the ultrasound appearance is not reliable, fine-needle aspiration or biopsy is almost always indicated when trying to establish a diagnosis and is reported to give the most accurate results in cases of gastric lymphoma.

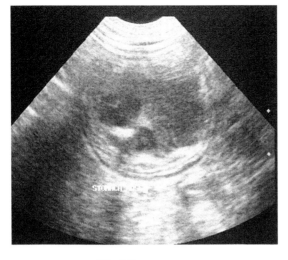

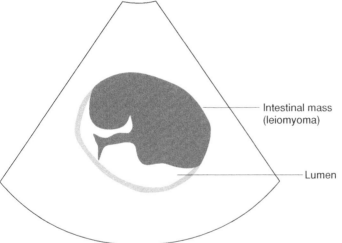

Intestinal mass
(leiomyoma)

Lumen

Figure 6.5 Gastric mass. In this case there is a large hypoechoic mass which appears to be occupying the gastric lumen. Sections of normal gastric wall can be seen. This localised mass is consistent with a leiomyoma or leiomyosarcoma.

Small and large intestinal neoplasia

The characteristic sonographic appearance of intestinal neoplasia is of a focal, asymmetrical thickening of the intestinal wall, with loss of layering and hypomotility (Figure 6.7 a & b). Erosion of the intestinal wall may be highlighted by hyperechoic foci of trapped gas at the luminal surface and surrounding inflammation. Focal gastro-intestinal tumours are generally easier to identify than diffuse neoplastic infiltrate, which may have a similar appearance to inflammatory

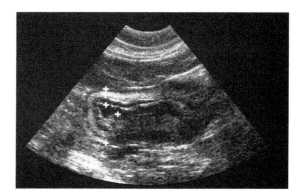

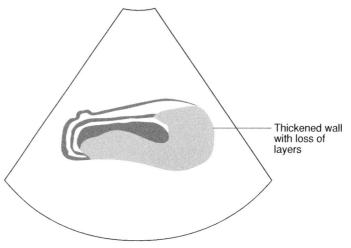

Thickened wall
with loss of
layers

Figure 6.6 Gastric mass. This hypoechoic intramural mass is typical of an intestinal neoplasm and has resulted in localised loss of wall layering. Fine-needle aspiration or biopsy is necessary for confirmation and to identify cell type. This appearance is more likely to be produced by lesions such as adenocarcinoma or lymphosarcoma than by leiomyoma or leiomyosarcoma. Gastric lymphoma was diagnosed.

conditions, especially in the case of lymphoma where layering of the intestine may be intact. In some cases, perforation of the intestinal wall occurs where neoplasia is present and this is accompanied by a local peritonitis and the attendant expected change such as increased brightness of the mesenteric tissue and local fluid accumulation.

It can sometimes be difficult to ascertain that a very large mass is associated with the intestine, especially if lying eccentrically to the bowel lumen. Gas within an abdominal mass is suggestive of intestinal involvement. Evidence of gastro-intestinal obstruction may be seen.

In the dog, adenocarcinoma is the most commonly seen intestinal neoplasm, followed by leiomyosarcoma and lymphoma. In the cat, apart from the more commonly seen

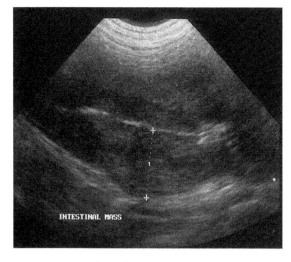

(a)

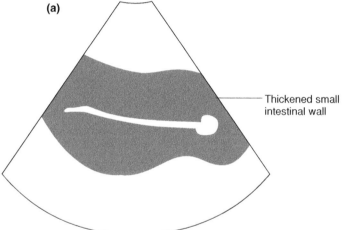

Thickened small intestinal wall

Figure 6.7 a & b Small intestinal neoplasia. The typical appearance of a hypoechoic intestinal mass is seen here in both longitudinal (a) and transverse (b) section. There is marked thickening of the intestinal wall and loss of layering.

lymphoma, leiomyosarcoma and mast cell tumours predominate. Adenocarcinoma lesions are usually hypoechoic and asymmetrical, whereas lymphoma tends to produce extensive symmetrical thickening of the small intestinal wall. Leiomyoma and leiomyosarcoma lesions have been reported to appear as solid masses which lie eccentrically in the bowel wall and often contain hypo- or anechoic cavities reflecting areas of necrosis. Leiomyosarcoma is most commonly seen in the jejunum and caecum and metastases frequently involve the liver and mesenteric lymph nodes.

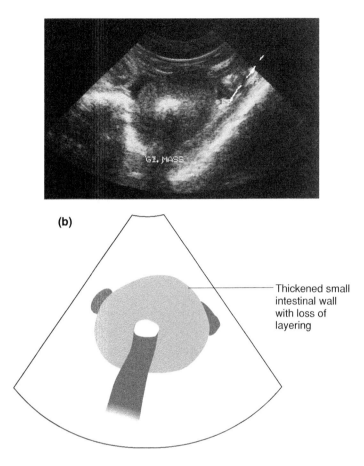

(b)

Thickened small intestinal wall with loss of layering

Figure 6.7 a & b
(*continued*)

Lymphoma is the commonest gastro-intestinal neoplasm in the cat and merits particular comment due to its characteristic features. Alimentary lymphoma can cause lymphoid infiltration of the stomach, intestine or mesenteric lymph nodes in cats of any age. The commonest sonographic finding is of a marked transmural thickening of the stomach or intestinal wall with partial or complete loss of layering, reduced wall echogenicity and localised hypomotility. In the small intestine, symmetrical thickening of the bowel wall can give a 'target lesion' appearance in transverse section. Other patterns of infiltration described as transmural-bulky, transmural-segmental, transmural-nodular or mucosal are less common manifestations. In the majority of cats, the lymphoma lesion is hypoechoic; however, in a small percentage of cats, mild increase in mucosal echogenicity with preservation of wall layering has been reported. This latter type of infiltration is more commonly seen with inflammatory bowel disease than with neoplasia. Most of the lymphoma lesions involve a large segment of the intestinal tract, making a differential diagnosis of inflammatory bowel disease and granulomatous enterocolitis necessary. In patients showing the localised segmental or nodular form of the disease, adenocarcinoma, mast cell tumour or severe localised inflammatory lesion should be considered. Involvement of the large intestine other than the ileocolic junction is uncommon in feline alimentary lymphoma.

Local lymph nodes may be enlarged, especially with gastric lesions. Lesions may be detectable sonographically in other organs including liver, kidneys, pancreas and the eye, and peritoneal effusion is seen in some cats. The presence of diffuse change in hepatic or renal echogenicity or localised lymphadenopathy gives weight to a provisional diagnosis of lymphosarcoma. Ultrasonography can be useful to monitor the response of lymphoma lesions to chemotherapy.

Other conditions

Intussusception

Intestinal intussusception is relatively common in young dogs and cats, where it tends to occur at the ileocolic junction. Predisposing causes include enteritis, foreign body, parasites or change of diet. In older animals, it may be secondary to neoplasia.

As the stomach, duodenum and large intestine can normally be identified, the anatomical position of an intussusception can often be determined by tracing the normal intestine adjacent to the lesion to one of these landmarks. In cross section, the intussusception appears as a circular lesion of concentric 'onion rings' which represent the multiple intestinal wall layers of the intussuscipiens within the intussusceptum. It is important to confirm the multi-layered appearance in two planes to avoid the possibility of misinterpreting the target appearance of some neoplastic lesions. The outer intussuscipiens tends to be oedematous and hypoechoic, whereas the inner intussusceptum is often hyperechoic (Figure 6.8).

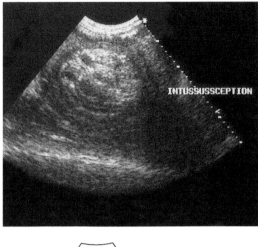

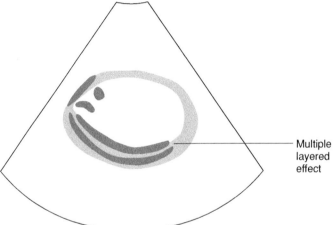

Figure 6.8 Intestinal intussusception. The typical, multi-layered appearance produced by an intussusception is shown here in transverse section. The lumen of the intussuscipiens is hyperechoic.

Multiple layered effect

Ultrasonography can determine the length of the intussusception, the patency of the bowel lumen and the presence of peritonitis or lymph node enlargement. Sections of intussuscepted bowel tend to be curved due to tension in the mesentery, which usually restricts their length to 12 cm or less. Lymph node enlargement may be present. Where necrosis of the intestinal wall occurs, loss of wall layering may be observed, as may free peritoneal fluid if peritonitis has developed. Since poor image quality can mimic loss of wall layering, findings suggestive of necrosis should be interpreted with care. A neoplastic lesion may be identified in conjunction with the intussusception. Intussusception involving the stomach has rarely been reported in animals. The sonographic appearance of gastrogastric intussusception, described in one dog, was of a mass in the fundus of the stomach with a 'target' appearance arising from the stomach wall layers. Gastroduodenal intussusception is rare but has been reported associated with duodenal ulceration.

Ileus

Accumulation of anechoic fluid within the intestine is always indicative of an abnormality. Mechanical ileus, which may be due to obstruction by foreign body or tumour, and paralytic (functional) ileus secondary to enteritis are possible causes of intestinal dilation. Acute mechanical ileus is usually associated with increased frequency of peristalsis, whereas this may be reduced or absent in more established cases. Mechanical ileus usually results in segmental dilation of bowel, while functional (paralytic) ileus, such as that associated with parvoviral enteritis or peritonitis, commonly leads to absence of peristaltic contraction and more uniform distension of the entire bowel. The aetiology of lack of intestinal peristalsis may not be identifiable sonographically. Markedly dilated fluid-filled intestine must be carefully differentiated from pyometra or paraprostatic cysts by tracing the dilated loops to their junction with normal bowel. Distended small intestine may also be mistaken for colon. The presence of active peristalsis helps to identify a loop of bowel as small intestine. The path of the colon is usually fixed and straighter than that of the small intestine.

Foreign body

Radio-opaque foreign bodies do not represent a great diagnostic challenge radiologically. However, the presence of a foreign body of soft tissue opacity may easily be overlooked on a radiograph. Sonography can be useful to detect a gastro-intestinal foreign body and assess for complications such as obstruction. It is, however, vital to remember that due to the presence of intraluminal gas, a foreign body can easily be overlooked on an abdominal scan alone and therefore sonography must always be preceded by survey radiographs.

The sonographic picture produced by a gastro-intestinal foreign body varies according to size, shape, material, surface characteristics and location of the object as well as the

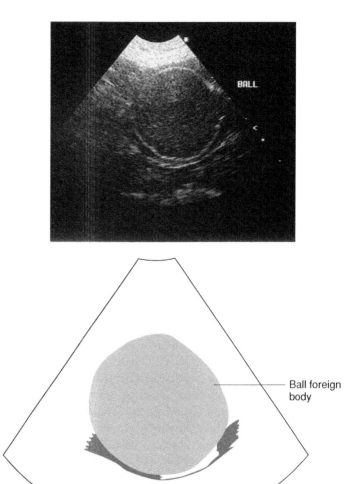

Figure 6.9 Intestinal foreign body. In this case a ball can be seen within the small intestine. Note the hyperechoic rim and the centre of low–moderate echogenicity. The appearance of a foreign body varies depending on its structure.

echogenicity of the surrounding luminal contents (Figure 6.9). Dense foreign bodies such as peach kernels, stones, or those containing gas, such as a ball, show a hyperechoic surface with distal acoustic shadowing. The acoustic shadow is often crisp and clean, similar to that observed with bone. Metallic foreign bodies are highly echogenic and cause characteristic reverberation and comet tail artefacts. Plastics often present a reflective double-surface layer. A rubber toy may produce acoustic shadowing without a hyperechoic near surface. Less dense objects may be difficult to identify sonographically.

A foreign body in the stomach or proximal duodenum usually leads to an abnormal increase in filling of the stomach and disturbance of peristalsis, which may increase or decrease. In the absence of luminal fluid, a gastric foreign body can be very difficult to identify. Gastric trichobezoars (fur balls) in the cat may appear as hyperechoic structures with a clear acoustic shadow, but have also been described as target lesions and as a heterogeneous, echogenic mass. Curvilinear shadowing within the lumen of the stomach is considered highly suggestive of a ball foreign body. Chronic gastric foreign body may lead to focal thickening of the gastric wall, local lymph node enlargement and pancreatitis. Some 'alternative' foodstuffs such as macaroni or water chestnuts can mimic a gastric foreign body, both sonographically and radiographically.

In the case of a small intestinal foreign body, increased filling of the intestinal loops is usual. An object can be more easily identified in an empty or fluid-filled loop of intestine than in the presence of gas and faecal material. Following the dilated loops of intestine will, in many cases, lead to the point of luminal obstruction. Where a mechanical obstruction is acute or subacute, waves of increased peristaltic activity with bi-directional flow of luminal fluid can usually be observed immediately proximal to the obstruction. Subacute or chronic obstruction results in atony giving an area void of peristalsis. Lack of peristalsis may also be caused by paralytic (functional) ileus secondary to inflammatory processes such as parvovirus enteritis or in association with recent abdominal surgery. Positive identification of a foreign body, enlarged lymph nodes or other differentiating feature is obviously helpful in such cases. A linear foreign body may cause a corrugated appearance in the small intestine due to increased/unproductive peristalsis. The affected small intestinal loops are usually dilated with fluid. Thickening of the intestinal wall may be seen if the wall becomes devitalised or where peritonitis develops, but wall layering is usually preserved.

Pancreas

Imaging procedure

The indications for sonography of the pancreas are similar to those for the gastro-intestinal tract and patient preparation is as for general abdomen – again, adequate starvation is essential otherwise gas in the adjacent bowel hinders visualisation. The pancreas is a V-shaped organ which lies in the right cranial quadrant of the abdomen and has both right and left limbs and a body. The right limb of the pancreas lies immediately dorsal to the duodenum and can be best imaged by scanning from the dependent side with the patient in right lateral recumbency. To localise the right limb of the pancreas, begin by placing the transducer to left of midline and angling the sound beam craniodorsally to identify the gastric fundus. Moving the transducer to the right, follow the path of the gastric antrum and pylorus to the descending duodenum. The duodenum and the pancreaticoduodenal vein, which runs parallel to the duodenum through the pancreatic lobe, are useful landmarks for the right limb of the pancreas (Figure 6.10). In the cat, the pancreatic duct is more commonly visualised than the vessel.

When significant quantities of gas are present in the stomach and duodenum, causing acoustic shadowing or reverberation artefacts, the right kidney may be used as a landmark. The right limb of the pancreas can be identified ventral to the kidney.

The left limb of the pancreas may not be clearly identifiable unless enlarged. It can be imaged from the left ventral abdominal wall using the spleen as an acoustic window. It lies dorsomedial to the spleen and caudal to the splenic vein in a triangle bound by the greater curvature of the stomach, the left kidney and the spleen. The portal and splenic veins are useful landmarks for the body and left lobe of the feline pancreas.

Normal appearance

In the normal dog, the pancreas is visualised as a region of high echogenicity relative to the renal cortex and liver parenchyma but is not well defined as it has a similar echogenicity to the surrounding mesentery and lacks capsular margination. Even with high frequency transducers the pancreatic margins are not well delineated from the surrounding structures. The normal feline pancreas is a smooth, homogeneous structure of similar echogenicity to the surrounding mesenteric fat, isoechoic or slightly hypoechoic to the liver and hypoechoic compared to the spleen.

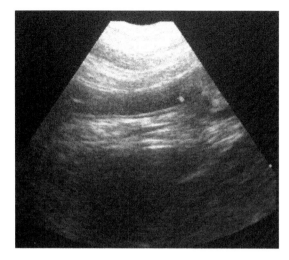

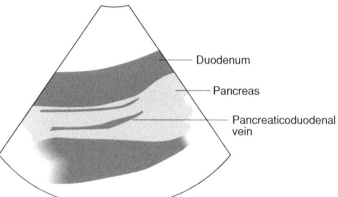

Duodenum

Pancreas

Pancreaticoduodenal vein

Figure 6.10
Pancreatic vessel. The duodenum and the pancreaticoduodenal vein are useful landmarks for the pancreas as seen here. Once the pancreas has been identified further evaluation of all sections is then possible.

Abnormal appearance

Pancreatitis

The sonographic changes associated with pancreatitis vary with severity and chronicity. Decreased echogenicity in acute pancreatitis reflect oedema, haemorrhage and necrosis. In cats, acute pancreatitis results in similar but less extensive changes to those in the dog.

Chronic pancreatitis may result in mineralisation and scarring which cause acoustic shadowing. The appearance of the inflamed pancreas can vary from an enlarged, homogeneous organ through an enlarged but ill defined hypoechoic

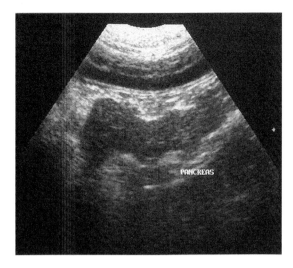

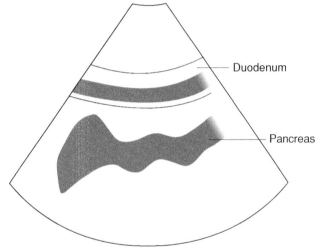

Figure 6.11
Resolving pancreatitis in a dog with subsequent biliary obstruction. Note the clear definition of the pancreas and the irregulariity of the borders with a generalised hypoechoic apppearance.

structure to a complex mass or multiple heterogeneous masses (Figure 6.11). The right lobe of the pancreas may move from its normal position dorsal or dorsomedial to the duodenum to lie dorsolaterally when markedly enlarged. In some cases, a solitary hypoechoic mass is seen in the pancreas, in others sonographic changes are mild or absent. A normal ultrasound examination of the pancreas does not rule out the possibility of pancreatitis.

Changes involving the adjacent stomach or duodenum may sometimes be the only sonographic findings in pancreatitis. The stomach or duodenum may be distended with fluid and show thickening of the wall and a lack of peristalsis due to functional ileus. The differential diagnosis of gastric and duodenal changes associated with pancreatitis includes focal peritonitis of other aetiology, gastroenteritis and gastro-intestinal neoplasia.

Changes in the pancreas may be accompanied by localised or generalised accumulation of peritoneal fluid. Focal fluid accumulation in the right cranial abdomen may be more likely with pancreatitis, whereas pancreatic neoplasia often results in more diffuse effusion. Severe pancreatitis however can also result in generalised peritoneal effusion.

It should be noted that pancreatitis, pancreatic abscess and pancreatic carcinoma can produce very similar sonographic abnormalities (Figure 6.12). Serial examination and fine-needle aspiration/biopsy can help differentiate these conditions. Pancreatitis tends to resolve on serial examination with successful treatment. In humans, ultrasonography of the pancreas has been used to confirm a diagnosis of acute pancreatitis and monitor its resolution or the development of sequelae such as pseudocysts.

Pancreatic pseudocysts are visualised as well defined anechoic lesions showing distal enhancement. The walls are generally thicker than those of renal cysts for example. Pancreatic necrosis can result in cavitary lesions which develop into pseudocysts. Pseudocysts associated with acute or chronic pancreatitis can resolve spontaneously without complication or may require intervention in the form of surgery or ultrasound-guided drainage.

The pancreatic duct may be dilated in some dogs with acute pancreatitis and can become as wide as the pancreaticoduodenal vein. A dilated pancreatic duct could be mistaken for a pseudocyst (Figure 6.13 a & b).

Mechanical obstruction or inflammation of the cholecystic duct due to a pancreatic lesion may lead to bile duct and gall bladder obstruction, causing post-hepatic jaundice. The presence of biliary obstruction does not help to differentiate between neoplastic and inflammatory processes. Sonographic changes associated with pancreatitis in the dog have been more frequently described than those in the cat, however similar findings may be seen in both species. In cases of feline pancreatitis, concurrent conditions such as hepatic lipidosis, cholangiohepatitis and inflammatory bowel disease may be associated with additional sonographic abnormalities.

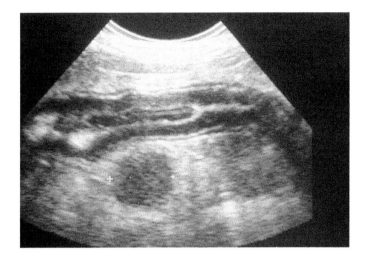

Figure 6.12
Pancreatic nodule in a dog. A hypoechoic nodule can be seen in the right limb of the pancreas. It appears well circumscribed and could represent an abscess, cyst/ pseudocyst or a tumour.

Pancreatic abscess

Pancreatic abscess is rare and is identified as a mass lesion in the right cranial abdomen with thick walls and hypoechoic contents, similar to other intra-abdominal abscesses. It is difficult to differentiate pancreatic abscess from necrosis or tumour. Diagnosis is by aspiration and culture, however pancreatic abscesses may be sterile.

Pancreatic neoplasia

Pancreatic tumours are rare. Fine-needle aspiration or biopsy is usually needed for confirmation. Adenocarcinoma is the

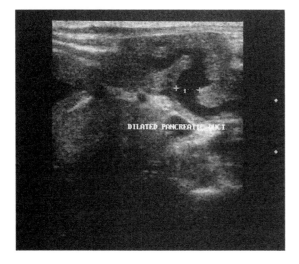

(a)

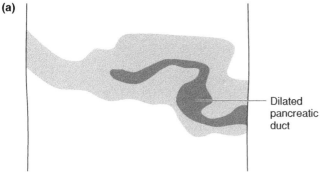

— Dilated pancreatic duct

Figure 6.13 a & b
Chronic pancreatitis in a cat. The dilated duct in the left limb of the pancreas can be seen. The hugely distended duct of the right limb is also seen, which in cross section could easily be mistaken for a cyst.

most common pancreatic neoplasm, seen in older animals. It often metastasises prior to clinical signs becoming evident and so may present at an advanced stage as a large mass in the region of the pancreas at the time of detection, often with dissemination through the abdominal cavity and peritoneal involvement (carcinomatosis). The common bile duct and pancreatic duct can become obstructed.

Islet cell tumours (insulinomata) are even less common than pancreatic carcinoma. Middle-aged dogs are most commonly affected, and there is a breed predisposition for the Boxer and Standard Poodle. Insulinoma of the pancreas can be detected sonographically as single or multiple well defined hypoechoic nodules or less commonly as a diffuse infiltrating process. Clinically significant lesions may be small and difficult to demonstrate sonographically. Metastasis is usually to regional lymph nodes and the liver. It helps in the

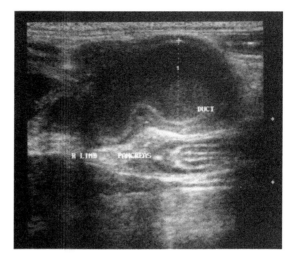

(b)

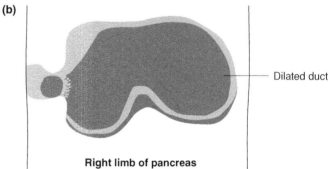

Dilated duct

Right limb of pancreas

Figure 6.13 a & b
(*continued*)

diagnosis of insulinoma if hyperglycaemia is present and an abnormal insulin/glucose ratio has been demonstrated, as sonographic changes can be more easily differentiated from those of acute pancreatitis. A negative scan does not rule out insulinoma as a diagnosis as there is a poor detection rate for this particular tumour.

Where there is a question of pancreatic neoplasia, the examination should include a search for lymph node enlargement and metastases to other abdominal organs. Enlargement of local lymph nodes has been reported to be suggestive of neoplasia, but is a non-specific finding, which may also accompany inflammatory disease of the pancreas.

Suggested reading

Biller, D. S., Partington, B. P., Miyabayashi, T., *et al.* (1994) Ultrasonographic Appearance of Chronic Hypertrophic Pyloric Gastropathy in
the Dog. In: *Veterinary Radiology and Ultrasound*, **35**, pp. 30–33.

Borgarelli, M., Biller, D. S., Goggin, J. M., *et al.* (1996) Part 1. Ultrasonographic Anatomy and Normal Findings. Part 2. Ultrasonographic Identification of Gastrointestinal Disease. Ultrasonographic Examination of
the Gastrointestinal System. In: *Veterinaria*, **10**, pp. 37–47.

Etue, S. M., Penninck, D. G., Labato, M. A., *et al.* (2001) Ultrasonography
of the Normal Feline Pancreas and Associated Anatomic Landmarks:
A Prospective Study of 20 Cats. In: *Veterinary Radiology and Ultrasound*, **42**, pp. 330–336.

Grooters, A. M., Biller, D. S., Ward, H., *et al.* (1994) Ultrasonographic
Appearance of Feline Alimentary Lymphoma. In: *Veterinary Radiology
and Ultrasound*, **35**, pp. 468–472.

Grooters, A. M., Miyabayashi, T. Biller, D. S., *et al.* (1994) Sonographic
Appearance of Uraemic Gastropathy in Four Dogs. In: *Veterinary
Radiology and Ultrasound*, **35**, pp. 35–40.

Kaser Hotz, B., Hauser, B. & Arnold, P. (1996) Ultrasonographic Findings Associated with Canine Gastric Neoplasia. In: Veterinary Radiology
and Ultrasound, 37, pp. 51–56.

Jergens, A. E. (1999) Inflammatory Bowel Disease: Current Perspectives.
In: *Veterinary Clinics of North America*, **29**, pp. 501–521.

Lamb, C. R. (1990) Abdominal Ultrasonography in Small Animals:
Intestinal Tract and Mesentery, Kidneys, Adrenal Glands, Uterus and
Prostate. In: *Journal of Small Animal Practice*, **31**, pp. 295–304.

Lamb, C. R. (1990) Abdominal Ultrasonography in Small Animals.
Examination of the Liver, Spleen and Pancreas. In: *Journal of Small
Animal Practice*, **31**, pp. 6–15.

Lamb, C. R. & Forster-van-Hijfte, M. (1994) Ultrasound Corner: Beware
the Gastric Pseudomass. In: *Veterinary Radiology and Ultrasound*, **35**,
pp. 398–399.

Lamb, C. R. & Grierson, J. (1999) Ultrasonographic Appearance of
Primary Gastric Neoplasia in 21 Dogs. In: *Journal of Small Animal
Practice*, **40**, pp. 211–215.

Lamb, C. R. & Mantis, P. (1998) Ultrasonographic Features of Intestinal
Intussusception in 10 Dogs. In: *Journal of Small Animal Practice*, **39**,
pp. 437–441.

Murtaugh, R. J., Herring, D. S., Jacobs, R. M., *et al.* (1985) Pancreatic
Ultrasonography in Dogs with Experimentally Induced acute
Pancreatitis. In: *Veterinary Radiology*, **26**, pp. 27–32.

Myres, N. C. & Pennick, D. G. (1994) Ultrasonographic Diagnosis of
Gastro-intestinal Smooth Muscle Tumours in the Dog. In: *Veterinary
Radiology and Ultrasound*, **35**, pp. 391–397.

Nyland, T. G., Mattoon, J. S., Herrgesell, E. J., *et al.* (2002) Pancreas.
In: *Small Animal Diagnostic Ultrasound*, 2nd edn, pp. 144–157. W. B.
Saunders Co., Philadelphia.

Penninck, D. G. (2002) Gastro-intestinal Tract, In: *Small Animal Diagnostic Ultrasound*, 2nd edn, pp. 207–230, W. B. Saunders Co.,
Philadelphia.

Penninck, D. G., Moore, A. S., Tidwell, A. S., *et al.* (1994) Ultrasonography
of Alimentary Lymphosarcoma in the Cat. In: *Veterinary Radiology and
Ultrasound*, **35**, p. 299.

Steiner, J. M. & Williams, D. A. (1999) Feline Exocrine Pancreatic Disorders. In: *Veterinary Clinics of North America*, **29**, pp. 551–575.

Tidwell, A. S. & Pennick, D. G. (1992) Ultrasonography of Gastrointestinal Foreign Bodies. In: *Veterinary Radiology and Ultrasound*, **33**, pp. 160–169.

Watson, P. J. (1997) Gastroduodenal Intussusception in a Young Dog. In: *Journal of Small Animal Practice*, **38**, pp. 163–167.

Willard, M. D. (1999) Feline Inflammatory Bowel Disease: A Review. In: *Journal of Feline Medicine and Surgery*, **1**, pp. 155–164.

Chapter 7

Urinary Tract

Johann Lang

Kidneys

Imaging technique

The superficial position of the kidneys means that they can be imaged from a ventral or lateral approach, and usually, even in large dogs, a 7.5 MHz transducer provides sufficient penetration to image the entire kidney and provide good resolution for a thorough evaluation of the renal structure. Because of their relatively caudal position, 7.5–10 MHz linear transducers are ideal for renal imaging in cats. If using a sector scanner, a stand-off pad may be required to obtain a good quality image of the near field in small or lean dogs and cats.

From the lateral aspect of the body wall images in the dorsal and transverse planes are obtained. For this purpose, a small area of hair is clipped and the site prepared with alcohol. On the left side this is just ventral to the sublumbar musculature caudal to the last rib and between the 11th and 12th intercostal space on the right. The animals are positioned in lateral recumbency and the kidneys can be imaged from the uppermost or the dependent side. After applying acoustic coupling gel, the transducer is held parallel to the long axis of the animal for longitudinal images and perpendicular to the spine for transverse images. It is often easier to locate the kidneys if one starts in the transverse plane moving the transducer slowly in a cranio-caudal direction. It is important to scan slowly through the entire kidney in both planes. Using the lateral approach, acoustic shadowing of the ribs can make it difficult to get a dorsal plane image of the right kidney. On the other hand, if using the lateral approach, examination of the kidneys with the animal in sternal recumbency or in the standing position is possible, which can be important in animals with large abdominal masses or ascites.

Sagittal plane images are obtained by imaging from the ventral body wall with the patient in dorsal recumbency and aligning the transducer parallel to the long axis. By rotating the transducer through 90°, transverse planes are obtained. Firm pressure must be applied to displace bowel loops, which are often located between the transducer and the kidney and this is particularly important in the deep-chested breeds. In dogs, the position of the right kidney within the rib cage and interference from overlying bowel loops can make it difficult to get a good quality image from the ventral body wall. The lateral approach is often preferred.

Normal appearance

Although the kidney has a similar appearance in both the dog and cat, some slight differences do exist. In cats, the kidneys are often more rounded than in the dog, where they are often bean shaped. The left kidney is located immediately caudal to the fundus of the stomach and caudomedial to the head of the spleen. When imaging the kidneys in dogs in dorsal recumbency, the spleen can sometimes be used as an acoustic window. The cranial pole of the right kidney sits in the renal fossa of the caudate lobe of the liver. The aorta and caudal vena cava (ventral and to the right of the aorta) are found between the kidneys.

The normal renal outline is smooth and well defined. Depending on the angle of the ultrasound beam, the capsule may be seen as a hyperechoic line and edge shadowing may be seen. In all planes, three distinct areas can be recognised: the renal cortex, renal medulla and renal sinus.

The renal sinus with its connective tissue and peripelvic fat is seen as a complex hyperechoic structure. While pyelectasia may be seen in some normal cases with no obvious cause it is more common for fluid not to remain within the renal pelvis.

The medulla, surrounding the renal sinus, is almost anechoic. In the sagittal and dorsal plane, it is divided into several sections by linear echogenicities, the recesses (or diverticula) and accompanying interlobar vessels. These traverse the medulla from the sinus to the cortex and are evenly spaced. Depending on the angle of the ultrasound beam and frequency of the transducer, these may generate acoustic shadowing and should not be mistaken for calculi. The interlobar and arcuate arteries between medulla and cortex are sometimes seen as short linear echogenicities. The renal crest, located between two sets of diverticula can be seen best on a mid-transverse plane (Figure 7.1 a–c).

The outermost layer is the renal cortex. Compared to the medulla, the cortex has a higher echogenicity, but is clearly hypoechoic compared to the spleen. If using a 5 MHz transducer the renal cortex appears to have a similar or slightly decreased echogenicity when compared to the liver. If higher frequency transducers are used it may appear more echogenic. Although this is a crude guide, marked changes in these relationships indicate possible pathology in the kidney, liver or spleen.

The normal ureters are not identified. In contrast, renal veins and arteries can be traced between kidney and aorta or caudal venal cava.

The kidney size can be assessed by measuring the length, width and height. From this, the renal volume can be calculated. In general sonography underestimates renal size but is sufficiently accurate to be clinically useful. In cats the anatomically measured length of the kidney is reported to be 3.8–4.4 cm, the width 2.7–3.1 cm and the height 2.0–2.5 cm. This measurement is close to the standards used for sonography. In cats, the renal size varies depending on whether the animals are intact or neutered. Neutered animals have smaller kidneys compared to intact animals, with no difference between the two sexes. In the dog, although a positive correlation between the size of the kidney and body weight is reported, the variation of kidney length in dogs with similar body weight is considerable. For clinical purposes calculating the volume of the kidney seems not to be necessary and measuring the length, width and height is adequate.

Table 7.1 Body weight versus kidney size in the normal dog.

Body weight (kg)	Lower limit (cm)	Upper limit (cm)
0–4	3.2	3.3
5–9	3.2	5.2
10–19	4.8	6.7
20–29	5.2	7.8
30–39	6.1	9.3
40–49	6.3	9.1
50–99	7.5	10.1

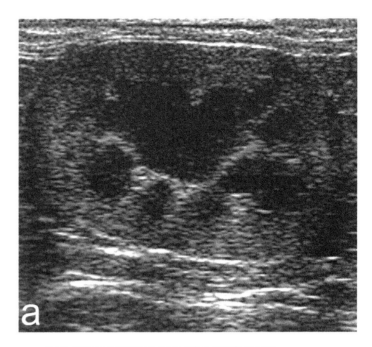

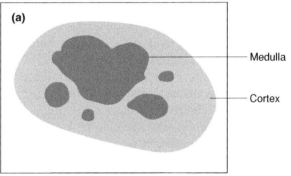

Figure 7.1 a–c
Sagittal (a), dorsal (b) and transverse (c) planes of a normal kidney in a cat. The renal cortex and the hypoechoic medulla are clearly distinguishable. The medulla is evenly spaced by the diverticula with the renal crest in the centre of the kidney.

Due to the increased size of the renal medulla, kidney size increases during diuresis. A mild degree of pyelectasia may be visible during intravenous fluid administration and this should not be interpreted as a pathological finding.

Abnormal appearance

Absence of a kidney

This may be the result of agenesis or previous nephrectomy. In some cases it may be difficult to localise or recognise a kidney sonographically. Large masses may produce

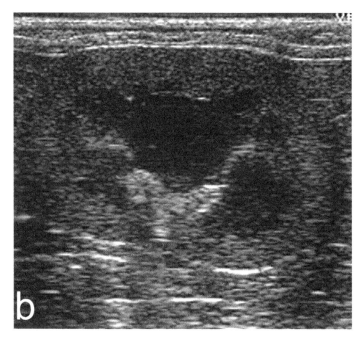

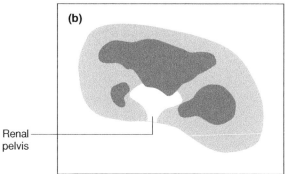

Figure 7.1 a–c
(b) The dorsal plane is perpendicular to the sagittal plane. The renal cortex has an intermediate echogenicity, the clearly hypoechoic medulla is separated by hyperechoic diverticula and interlobar vessels. The hilar region containing the renal sinus and peripelvic fat has a high echogenicity.

displacement or severely hypoplastic or end-stage kidneys with destroyed internal architecture may be challenging for the examiner to identify. Tracing the renal artery with colour Doppler from the aorta distally can be helpful in finding a small kidney not detected by the standard examination technique.

Focal parenchymal abnormalities

In general, focal abnormalities are more easily identified than diffuse renal disease. Depending on the size of the animal, the transducer used and type of the abnormality, even very small

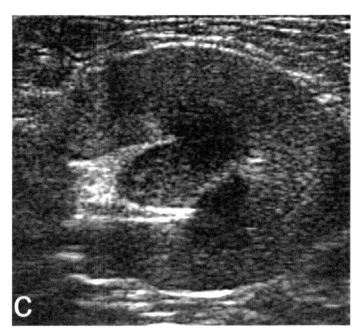

Figure 7.1 a–c (c)
In this mid-transverse plane, the renal cortex, the hypoechoic medulla and the renal sinus are demonstrated. The pelvis consists of a faint hypoechoic line, bordered by two hyperechoic lines.

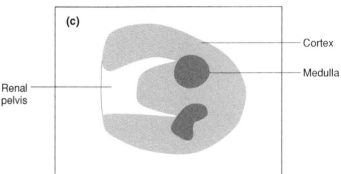

focal lesions can be seen. Cysts are relatively easy to detect. Smaller, solid lesions, which do not distort the renal contour or the internal architecture, may be more difficult to detect and require a thorough examination of the kidney in multiple planes. The sonographic properties of solid lesions are non-specific and do not allow a definitive diagnosis to be made.

Renal cysts

Cysts may be solitary or multiple and may be uni- or bilateral. Sonographically, cysts are usually round or ovoid structures with a smooth, thin and well defined wall and anechoic

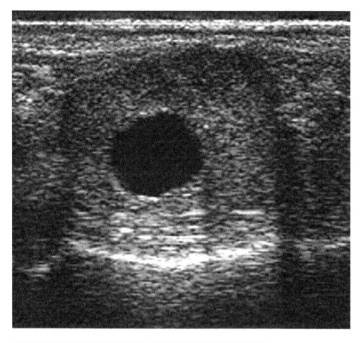

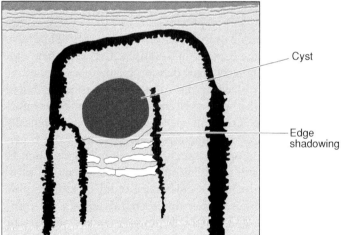

Figure 7.2 Renal cyst. Transverse plane of the caudal pole of a kidney with a cyst: the kidney has an irregular border and contains an anechoic round structure with a sharply demarcated far wall border. There is acoustic enhancement distant to the lesion and edge shadowing at the lateral borders of the cyst and kidney.

Cyst

Edge shadowing

content (Figure 7.2). The far wall is usually sharply demarcated and distant acoustic enhancement is seen. The latter two features are helpful for distinguishing solid but hypoechoic lesions, such as lymphoma, from cysts. The latter remain anechoic if the gain settings of the machine are increased, whereas hypoechoic lesions are seen to have internal structure. Cysts may show edge shadowing and slice-thickness artefacts, mimicking the presence of sediment. In superficial cysts, assessment of the near wall may be difficult due to reverberation artefact. Large or multiple cysts often distort the contour of the kidney and may cause displacement and distortion of the collecting system. Complicated cysts may have thick or irregular walls, may be septate and often contain multiple corpuscular echoes.

Cysts may be heritable or secondary to chronic nephropathy. Hereditary forms of polycystic renal disease have been described in Persian and other long-haired cats as well as Cairn terriers. Occasionally these cysts are associated with pancreatic or hepatic cysts. Occasionally, multiple, very small cysts are seen in cats with polycystic kidney disease and this may lead to a coarse echotexture with diffusely increased echogenicity.

Differential diagnoses for complicated cysts must include renal abscess, haematoma, granuloma and cystic neoplasia. These often exhibit many, but only rarely all, features of a simple cyst. Cysts in cystadenoma carcinomas of the kidneys – associated with dermatofibrosis in female German Shepherd dogs – usually have a thick, irregular wall and contain echogenic debris. Renal abscesses are rare in the dog and cat but are seen as complex masses of mixed echogenicity containing anechoic or hyperechoic components. They have many sonographic features of a complicated cyst, often with irregular walls and echogenic debris. Haematomas may occur in animals with bleeding disorders or after trauma. These can be associated with perirenal or subcapsular haemorrhage or rupture of the renal pelvis or ureter. Sonographically it is not possible to distinguish acute bleeding from urine, because both will present as anechoic fluid accumulation in the area of the kidney. Avulsion of the kidney requires careful examination using Doppler ultrasound or radiographic contrast procedures. Other differential diagnoses for complex masses are granulomas, acute infarcts and primary or metastatic tumours. History, clinical examination and analysis of blood and urine samples will often lead to the correct diagnosis. However, in many cases only invasive procedures such as fine-needle aspiration or biopsy will be diagnostic.

Renal neoplasia

Most solid kidney masses are neoplastic in origin. They may present as hypoechoic, isoechoic or hyperechoic lesions (Figure 7.3). The echogenicity or the echotexture is not

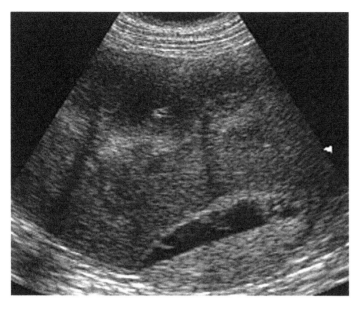

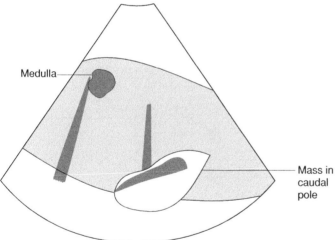

Figure 7.3 Large complex mass in the caudal pole of the left kidney in a dog. The poorly defined mass is slightly hyperechoic compared to the normal parenchyma. At the border of this mass there is a cyst-like lesion (complicated cyst) with an irregular hyperechoic wall and hyperechoic sediment. Differential diagnoses include haematoma, abscess formation, tumour and granuloma. In this case, the diagnosis was haematoma of unknown origin.

characteristic for a specific tumour type. Lymphoma nodules often present as uniformly hypoechoic lesions, but in contrast to a cyst the distal wall is not well demarcated, there is no distant enhancement and increasing the gain or using a higher frequency transducer will increase the echogenicity. Differential diagnoses of solid kidney masses include lymphoma, cystadenocarcinoma, sarcomas and most metastatic tumours (Figure 7.4 a & b). Isoechoic masses may only be recognised if the renal contour and/or internal architecture

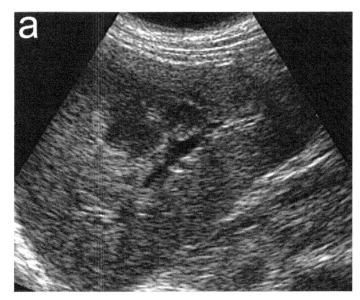

Figure 7.4a
Hyperechoic renal mass in a dog with renal lymphosarcoma – sagittal plane. The cranial pole of the kidney is enlarged and the irregularly defined mass is hyperechoic to the normal parenchyma. The normally hypoechoic medulla has been replaced by isoechoic tissue. The renal pelvis is enlarged and has a straight shape with rounded edges. Differential diagnoses include other renal tumours.

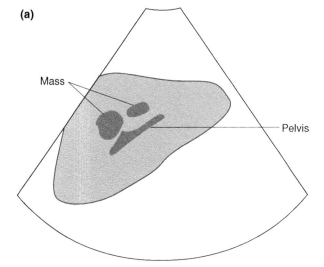

is distorted. Hyperechoic masses are relatively rare but seem to be associated with well vascularised tumours. Differential diagnoses include haemangiosarcoma, haemangioma, metastatic thyroid carcinoma and chondrosarcoma. Occasionally, non-neoplastic lesions may present as solid masses as well. The final diagnosis is usually based on history, laboratory work, and fine-needle aspiration or core biopsy. Parenchymal mineralisation, fibrosis, gas and chronic renal

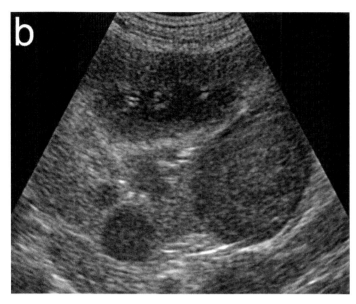

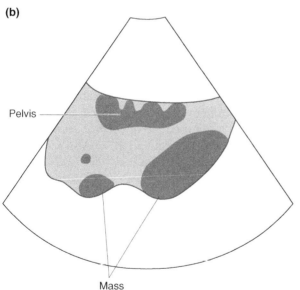

(b)

Pelvis

Mass

Figure 7.4b
Solid masses in the
left kidney in a dog –
dorsal plane. The
masses of differing
sizes are hypoechoic
to the renal cortex and
protrude from the
normal border of the
kidney. The large mass
in the caudal pole
is distorting the
normal architecture.
Differential diagnoses
include primary and
metastatic renal
tumour, focal renal
lymphosarcoma and
granuloma (rare).
The pattern is not
characteristic of a
specific tumour type
and requires biopsy.

infarcts may lead to hyperechoic areas without mass effect.
Acute infarcts usually present as mass-like lesions with
decreased or mixed echogenicity and chronic infarcts as
triangular or wedge-shaped lesions with the tip at the
corticomedullary junction. The renal contour in the area of
an infarct may be flattened or indented.

Diffuse parenchymal abnormality

Increased cortical echogenicity

Diffuse renal disease is difficult to assess sonographically. Changes are often non-specific and a normal sonographic examination does not exclude renal disease. However, ultrasound examination of the kidney is helpful in the differentiation of acute and chronic renal disease where there is acute onset of clinical signs.

Acute glomerulonephritis, interstitial nephritis, amyloidosis, diffuse neoplastic infiltrate (e.g. lymphoma), acute tubular necrosis or nephrosis (e.g. ethylene glycol toxicity) and metastatic neoplasia, such as squamous cell carcinoma and mast cell tumour, may all lead to increased echogenicity of the renal cortex (Figure 7.5).

Feline infectious peritonitis should also be considered in cats where other findings are suggestive. The kidneys are often unilaterally or bilaterally enlarged. Increased echogenicity of the renal cortex with loss of corticomedullary differentiation has been described in polycystic renal disease. In older, castrated male cats without renal dysfunction, cortical echogenicity may be increased due to fat vacuoles in the epithelium of the proximal cortical tubules. In both species chronic inflammatory renal disease and end-stage kidneys will lead to an increase in cortical echogenicity and poor corticomedullary differentiation. End-stage kidneys are usually small and irregular. Fibrosis will lead to diffusely increased echogenicity with a loss of the corticomedullary differentiation and internal architecture (Figure 7.6).

Increased echogenicity of the cortex may be associated with abnormalities of the corticomedullary junction. In hypercalcaemic nephropathy and acute tubular nephrosis or necrosis as result of ethylene glycol poisoning, a hyperechoic rim at the corticomedullary junction has been described. Chronic hypercalcaemia will eventually lead to severe renal damage with calcification of the basement membrane of the Bowman's capsule and adjacent renal tubules. In cases with hypercalcaemic nephropathy, the hyperechoic corticomedullary band is reported to be a poor prognostic sign. Possible causes include lymphoma, myeloma and adenocarcinoma of the anal sac. Renal disease without hypercalcaemia may also lead to the renal medullary rim sign. The renal medullary rim sign has been described in normal animals and seems

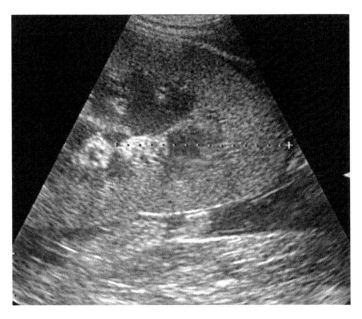

(a)

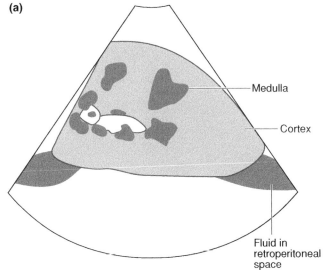

Medulla

Cortex

Fluid in
retroperitoneal
space

Figure 7.5 a & b
Acute nephritis in a 10-
month-old dog (25 kg)
with leptospirosis. Both
kidneys are enlarged,
measuring between
9.7 and 10 cm. Around
the left kidney there is
free fluid in the
retroperitoneal space.
The kidney is well
displayed. Compared
to the liver, the cortex
of the right kidney is
hyperechoic. The
cortex appears
thickened and the
corticomedullary
junction is well
preserved.

to be associated with mineral deposits in the lumen of the
proximal tubules but the cause remains unclear (Figure 7.7).

Decreased cortical echogenicity

Decreased echogenicity of the renal cortex has been described as a result of necrosis and with lymphoma infiltrate

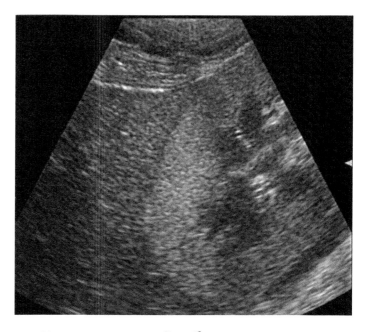

(b)

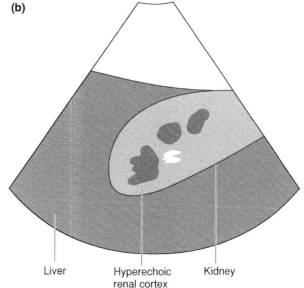

Figure 7.5 a & b
(*continued*)

Liver   Hyperechoic   Kidney
            renal cortex

which may also present with multiple, small hypoechoic nodules or masses.

In all cases, a definitive diagnosis cannot be made on the basis of the ultrasound alone and other procedures such as renal biopsy may be required.

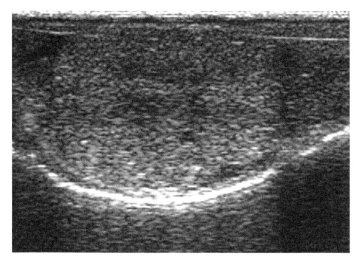

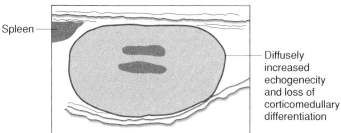

Spleen

Diffusely
increased
echogenecity
and loss of
corticomedullary
differentiation

Figure 7.6 End stage renal disease in a cat. Compared to the spleen, the kidney shows a diffusely increased echogenicity with loss of the corticomedullary definition caused by the increased echogenicity of the medulla. The kidney is small and has an irregular cranial border.

Collecting system, pelvis and ureters

Hydronephrosis

In normal animals, the renal pelvis does not retain fluid and is not visible sonographically. The most commonly seen abnormality of the collecting system, pelvis and ureters is dilation, and ultrasound is a sensitive technique for investigating the potential causes. Differential diagnoses include congenital anomaly, ureteric obstruction, pyelonephritis, and diuresis following administration of intravenous fluids or diuretic.

Cases with mild pyelectasia may be difficult to detect and careful examination is required. Differentiation of a mildly dilated renal pelvis from the renal vessels can be made by tracing the renal veins and arteries using colour-flow Doppler ultrasound. Scanning in the transverse plane is very helpful and may reveal the hypoechoic V-shaped dilated renal pelvis surrounding the renal crest, and a dilated ureter extending medially may be seen. In mild cases,

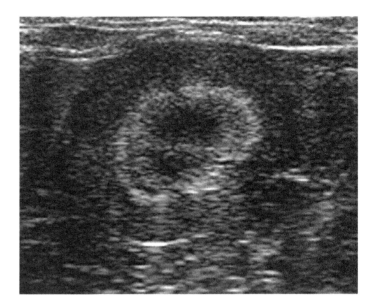

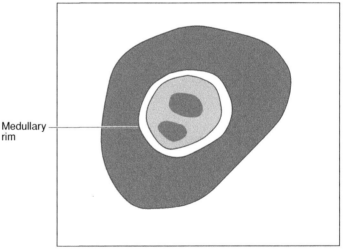

Figure 7.7 Renal medullary rim sign in a clinically normal cat. This finding is non-specific, and can be found in clinically normal dogs and cats, as well as those with hypercalcaemic nephropathy and other pathological conditions.

Medullary rim

the renal architecture remains normal. If the dilation increases, the diagnosis is more easily confirmed. The normally hyperechoic structures of the peripelvic fat gradually disappear and the pelvic diverticula and proximal ureter become more dilated. This specific appearance is also helpful in differentiating a dilated renal pelvis from a renal cyst. With increasing amounts of fluid, the normal renal architecture disappears as the parenchyma is compressed. Severe hydronephrosis is most often associated with long-standing and severe ureteral obstruction and the kidney is seen as a round or ovoid anechoic sac. A thin rim of parenchyma and several hyperechoic bands extending from the hilus to the capsule are typical findings. In any patient with hydronephrosis, the ureter must be examined thoroughly. While it is relatively easy to recognise a dilated ureter in the area of the kidney and close to the trigone region of the bladder, it may be very difficult in the middle section. The dilated ureter is often tortuous and peristalsis, if seen, is helpful for differentiating the ureter from blood vessels. The bladder neck must always be carefully examined because tumours of the bladder, prostate and urethra may extend into the trigone region, obstructing the ureters and resulting in uni- or bilateral hydronephrosis. Congenital anomalies such as ectopic ureters and ureteroceles are common causes of hydronephrosis. Ureteral obstruction caused by intrinsic or extrinsic tumour or inflammation and ureteral calculi may occasionally be seen as well.

Acute pyelonephritis may or may not cause dilation of the renal pelvis but in more chronic cases this may be mild to moderate and may be uni- or bilateral (Figure 7.8 a & b). A hyperechoic line in the wall of the pelvis, seen in the transverse plane, can be a sign of acute pyelonephritis. In chronic cases, distortion of the diverticula and pelvis, increased echogenicity with poor corticomedullary differentiation, and decreased renal size with irregular kidney contour can be seen.

Renal calculi

Renal calculi are usually easy to detect sonographically (Figure 7.9). Both radiopaque and radiolucent renal calculi are intensely hyperechoic, with clean acoustic shadowing. Acoustic shadowing is an important feature for differentiating calculi from blood clots, as the latter, although hyperechoic, do not produce an acoustic shadow and their ultrasound appearance will change with time. In questionable cases, the examination can be repeated a few days later. Calculi produce maximal shadowing if the highest possible transducer frequency is chosen and the ultrasound beam is directed perpendicular to the lesion in question, which should be located within the focal zone of the transducer. Calculi are especially easy to detect if they are associated with dilation of the renal pelvis. Small calculi, especially if located within the renal parenchyma, may be difficult to differentiate from the shadowing produced by the walls of the diverticula.

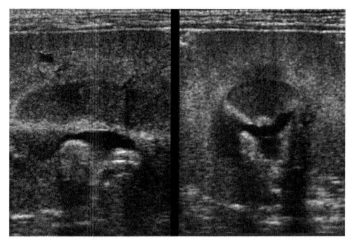

Figure 7.8 a & b
Dorsal and transverse images of the kidney in a dog with pyelonephritis. There is mild dilatation of the renal pelvis. The overall architecture of the kidney is normal. however the renal cortex appears broad and hyperechoic. In the renal cortex a small cyst is present.

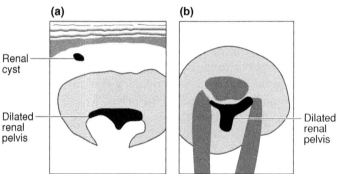

Masses of inflammatory or neoplastic origin may have a variable echogenicity and often lead to distortion of the collecting system and asymmetric pelvic dilatation. In questionable cases intravenous urography can be helpful to distinguish between parenchymal calcification and calculi, blood clots or other masses. The latter produce distortion of the collecting system, filling defects and are located centrally.

Perinephric fluid accumulation

Subcapsular or extracapsular fluid accumulation has been described in cats. These pseudocysts are not lined by an epithelium, can be very large and often are palpable masses. Sonographically, the kidneys are surrounded by encapsulated anechoic fluid. The kidney size, architecture and function are usually normal. Since underlying disease processes like trauma with ruptured kidney, renal pelvis or ureter, infection (FIP), toxicity or tumours also may cause subcapsular

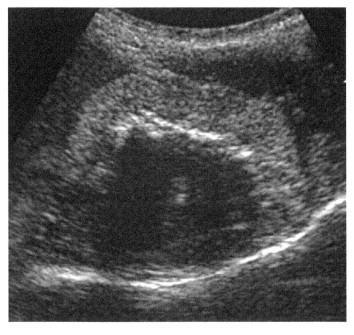

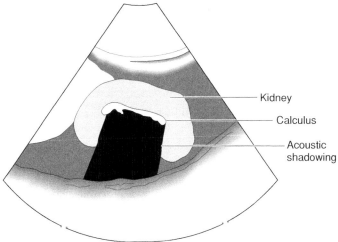

Kidney

Calculus

Acoustic
shadowing

Figure 7.9 Large renal calculus in a dog with chronic pyelonephritis. Compared with the spleen, the renal cortex is hyperechoic. The calculus (arrows) presents as a hyperechoic structure with shadowing distant to it. Small pelvic calculi can be located anywhere, large calculi are most often located centrally.

or extracapsular fluid accumulation, aspiration of fluid or renal biopsy for analysis is required.

Bladder

Imaging procedure

The superficial position of the urinary bladder and the inherent contrast produced by the anechoic urine makes it ideal for ultrasound examination. Because identification of the empty bladder is difficult and wall thickness is determined by the degree of distension, it is recommended that the bladder be moderately full for the examination. Complete distension is not necessary or helpful. Ischaemia, haemorrhage, cystitis and rupture are potential risks, and maximum distension also may mask subtle abnormalities of the bladder wall.

The bladder can be seen most easily with the animal in dorsal recumbency and the transducer positioned at the ventral or ventrolateral aspect of the caudal abdominal wall. While a 5.0–10 MHz sector, convex or microconvex transducer is suitable for the examination, high frequency linear transducers (7.5–10 MHz) or stand-off pads are required to evaluate the ventral bladder wall. The type and frequency of the transducer is determined by the position of the bladder (abdominal or pelvic), patient size and the depth, penetration and resolution required. Examination is made in both longitudinal and transverse planes from the cranial pole to the trigone and the proximal urethra. Depending on the position of the bladder, the proximal part of the urethra, e.g. the prostatic part in male dogs, can be evaluated as well. The examination should include evaluation of the regional lymph nodes. Bladder size and shape are assessed as well as the appearance of the bladder wall including layering, thickness and mucosal surface. The appearance of the content is also important.

Normal appearance

While usually intra-abdominal in location, the bladder may occasionally be found in an intrapelvic position. It usually has a round or ovoid appearance but this depends on the degree of distension, pressure from surrounding structures, such as colon or an adjacent mass, and possible bladder pathology. If the ultrasound beam is perpendicular to the surface of the bladder, the characteristic appearance of the bladder wall is of two distinct thin hyperechoic lines separated by a hypoechoic layer. The thickness of the normal bladder increases with body weight and depends on the degree of distension. In the near-empty bladder the mean wall thickness was measured to be 2.3 +/– 0.43 mm, when moderately distended (4 ml/kg) it was 1.4 +/– 0.28 mm. If

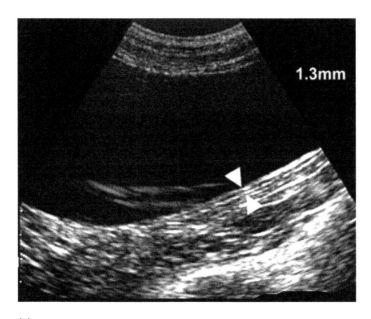

(a)

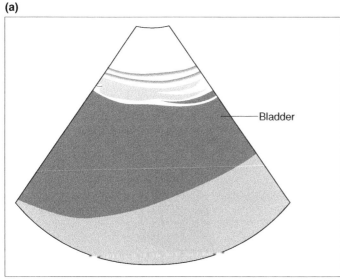

Bladder

Figure 7.10a
(a) Sagittal and (b) transverse planes of a normal bladder: note the normal layering and thickness (1.3 mm) of the moderately distended bladder. On the image in the transverse plane, the colon, containing highly echogenic material which produces an acoustic shadow, is pressing into the bladder. This should not be mistaken for a urinary calculus.

distended, the mucosal surface is smooth, whereas if empty, folding of the mucosa causes an irregular undulating surface (Figure 7.10 a & b). The content is normally anechoic, but floating corpuscular echoes occasionally occur in patients without urinary tract disease.

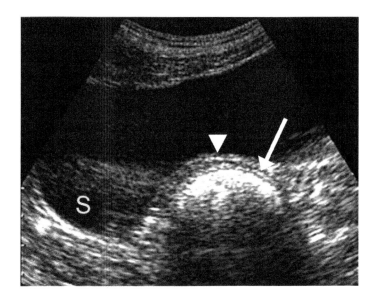

(b)

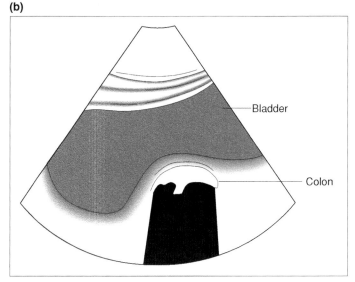

Figure 7.10b
Note the walls of the bladder (arrows) and the colon (arrow heads) covering the 'pseudo stone'. The echogenic 'bands' in the bladder are caused by side lobe artefacts. This is also termed pseudo sludge.

Abnormal appearance

Bladder neoplasia

Thickening of the bladder wall is most commonly associated with neoplastic or inflammatory infiltration. The most common tumour of the bladder wall is transitional cell carcinoma, but other epithelial and mesenchymal tumours such as leiomyoma, leiomyosarcoma, fibrosarcoma and lymphoma

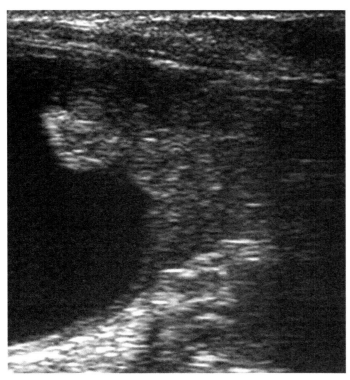

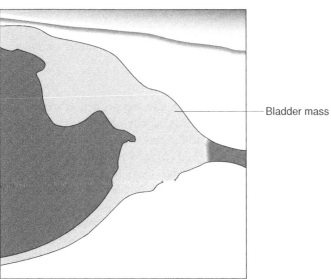

Bladder mass

Figure 7.11 Sagittal view of the trigone area in a cat with transitional cell carcinoma. A single, large sessile mass with an irregular surface is seen projecting into the bladder lumen. There is invasion of the bladder wall (arrows). Complications of tumours at this site include obstruction of the ureters and the urethra.

can also occur. Transitional cell carcinoma may result in one of the four sonographic patterns:

1 single sessile mass with or without invasion of the wall (Figure 7.11)
2 multiple sessile masses
3 a single pedunculated mass and
4 irregular bladder wall with the shape varying from regular nodules to very irregularly shaped masses.

The echogenicity is usually reduced compared with the normal bladder wall and in some cases may have a more complex appearance. The transition between tumour and normal bladder wall is usually abrupt but where there is infiltration of the wall this may be less clear. Transitional cell carcinomas are most often located in the area of the trigone, dorsal wall and proximal urethra but may also be seen in the other parts of the bladder.

Hydronephrosis and hydroureter may be associated with tumours involving the trigone. Tumours located in the urethra cannot be fully assessed using sonography and in these cases a urethrogram or urethroscopy are required to evaluate the whole length of the urethra.

Fine-needle aspirate or catheter biopsy and evaluation of the sublumbar region for lymphadenopathy may enable a diagnosis to be confirmed as inflammatory polyps, blood clots, cystitis and calculi may 'mimic' a bladder tumour.

Cystitis

Cystitis is the most common disease process involving the urinary bladder. Acute cystitis usually causes no sonographic abnormalities. Long-standing and severe cystitis often leads to diffuse bladder wall thickening, with a hyperechoic wall and irregular mucosal surface, and is usually more pronounced cranioventrally but may involve the entire bladder wall in severe cases (Figure 7.12). Polypoid cystitis usually presents as wall thickening with multiple small nodules protruding into the bladder lumen, but large polyps may be seen as pedunculated masses. Since bladder wall neoplasia is more common than polypoid cystitis, the diagnosis has to be confirmed with biopsy.

Other abnormalities

Other abnormalities of the bladder wall include mural haematomas and diffuse haemorrhage associated with bleeding

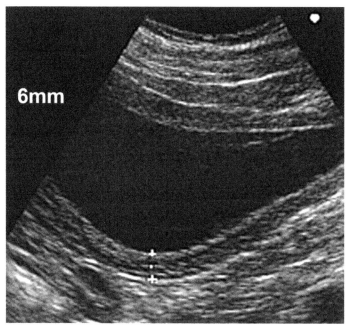

6mm

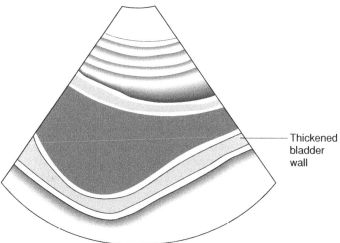

Thickened
bladder
wall

Figure 7.12 Sagittal
plane images of a dog
with a chronic lower
urinary tract infection:
The entire wall of this
moderately distended
bladder is thickened
(6 mm). In mild cases,
there is often no
thickening or only
thickening of the
ventral bladder wall. In
these cases, a linear
transducer or a stand-
off pad can be helpful.

disorders. Diffuse hyperechoic wall thickening associated with echogenic luminal content is the predominant
feature of haematuria. Patent urachal diverticula (congenital or acquired) are difficult to assess sonographically due
to their cranioventral location. Positive or double-contrast
cystography is more sensitive. A diverticulum may be suspected if the bladder has an unusually pointed appearance

but only rarely can a fluid-filled structure extending from the bladder wall can be seen. Diverticula may predispose to recurrent bladder infection but may also be the result of inflammatory disease. Bladder wall rupture may be difficult to assess sonographically. A ruptured bladder may present with free abdominal fluid and wall thickening, however, sonography combined with catheterisation of the bladder and injection of saline solution may show the site of the rupture.

Ectopic ureters and ureteroceles associated with hydroureter and hydronephrosis may also be seen. A ureterocele is a congenital stenosis of the opening of a ureter resulting in dilatation. They present as smooth and well defined cystic structures in the area of the trigone and in real time their size changes depending on the peristalsis of the ureter. Dilated ectopic ureters may be seen entering the bladder wall at the normal anatomical site or passing the wall parallel to it and opening into the urethra, or into the vagina, which is difficult to detect sonographically. Radiographic contrast studies or endoscopy are often required to confirm the diagnosis.

Bladder content

Many of the conditions described above are also associated with abnormal luminal content. Blood clots may be associated with tumour, infection, trauma and bleeding disorders. They are usually irregularly shaped masses and tend to settle on the dependent side of the bladder. While smaller clots are hyperechoic without distant shadowing, larger clots tend to be more hypoechoic. Large and/or adherent blood clots are less mobile and can mimic mural lesions. Positional studies, agitation of the transducer, and injection of additional saline solution may resuspend the clots and often help to determine the nature of the lesion.

Except for single, very small stones, cystic calculi are easy to detect sonographically where they present as hyperechoic lesions with shadowing in the dependent portion of the bladder (Figure 7.13). This appearance is regardless of their radiopacity. The amount of shadowing depends on the size of the calculus, the composition, the transducer frequency used, and whether the soundbeam is directed perpendicular to the surface. With positional studies (where the patient position is changed so that the dependent region of the

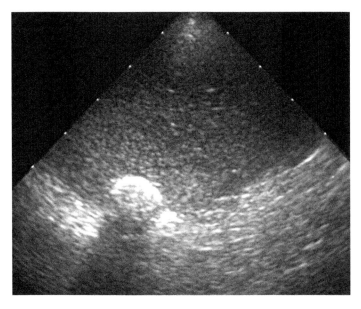

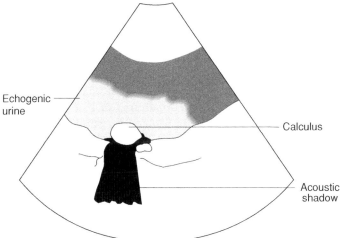

Echogenic urine

Calculus

Acoustic shadow

Figure 7.13 Highly echogenic cellular urine is present in this dog with acute haemorrhage. Because of the increased echogenicity of the urine, the bladder wall is difficult to assess. A strongly hyperechoic calculus with acoustic shadowing is also present.

bladder changes) most calculi migrate to the dependent part of the bladder. Occasionally, but only rarely, they may adhere to the bladder wall and can be mistaken for bladder wall calcification. Hyperechoic sediment with shadowing also occurs. When agitated, sediment suspends easily, leading to corpuscular echogenicities with no distinct calculi distinguishable. Floating echogenicities without shadowing may be seen where the urine contains cellular debris, blood or fibrin (hyperechoic strands). Gas bubbles also present as hyperechoic floating foci with shadowing and are frequently seen following bladder catheterisation. In contrast to sediment, they tend to rise to the top of the bladder. Intramural gas produces a highly echogenic bladder wall with acoustic shadowing and it may be very difficult to identify the bladder.

Prostate

Imaging procedure

Prostatic disease is rare in the cat and there are few indications for the ultrasonographic examination of this organ. The imaging technique described applies to the dog but if necessary may be applied to the cat.

Ultrasonographic examination of the prostate gland may be performed by rectal or trans-abdominal routes. The rectal approach has the advantage of allowing the prostate to be imaged even when it lies in an intrapelvic position, but a transducer designed specifically for rectal work is necessary. A trans-abdominal approach is in most instances satisfactory and no specialised transducer is required.

The examination should be performed with the bladder moderately distended. A full bladder acts as an easily recognisable landmark and displaces gas-filled small intestine from the caudal abdomen. The dog should be placed in dorsal or lateral recumbency and a small area of hair clipped on one side of the prepuce just in front of the pubic brim. After routine skin preparation, the transducer should be placed perpendicular to the skin surface with the plane of the ultrasound beam, approximately parallel to the prepuce. Once the bladder has been identified it is possible to move caudally towards the neck of the bladder and thence to the prostate. If the prostate lies partly or wholly within the pelvic canal it may be necessary to angle the transducer caudally under the pubic rim. Alternatively, a gloved finger may be placed per rectum and the prostate pushed gently forward. Occasionally in immature dogs or dogs neutered at an early age, it may prove difficult to image the prostate but in such cases disease is unlikely. Once the prostate has been identified in longitudinal section a sweep from side to side should be made. The transducer should then be rotated through 90° to achieve a transverse section and a sweep made from one end of the gland to the other. In this way a thorough examination of the entire gland can be made. It may on occasions be helpful to place an air- or fluid-filled urethral

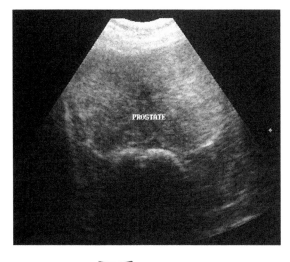

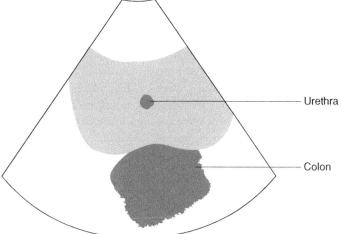

Urethra

Colon

Figure 7.14   Normal transverse image of the prostate. Note the symmetrical bilobed appearance and the hypoechoic spot centrally representing the intraprostatic urethra. Note also the hyperechoic rim of the colon deep to the prostate.

catheter *in situ* to enable an assessment of prostatic symmetry to be made.

Normal appearance

The normal prostate in the dog is smooth in outline and fairly well circumscribed. It varies in shape from spherical to clearly bilobed or pear-shaped (Figure 7.14). The prostatic parenchyma is normally moderately echogenic with a coarse but even texture throughout. Linear echogenic streaks may be detected running longitudinally through the middle of

the gland. This is the 'hilar echo' and is thought to represent peri-urethral fibrous tissue. The prostatic urethra may
be seen running through the parenchyma as a fine, linear
anechoic structure.

Variations in the size and ultrasonographic appearance of
the normal prostate according to age and history of neuter-
ing have yet to be defined.

Abnormal appearance

The appearance of prostatic abnormality may be divided
into focal and diffuse parenchymal lesions and paraprostatic.
Again, it is very important to note that it is not possible to
make a histological diagnosis based on the ultrasound features alone.

Focal parenchymal lesions

Focal disturbances in the normal, even echotexture of the prostate should be carefully evaluated. The number of lesions,
their size and shape, the clarity of their outline and their
echogenicity should all be noted. It is important to determine whether lesions are intra- or paraprostatic.

The commonest focal lesions identified on ultrasonographic examination of the prostate are intraprostatic cysts.
Small cysts (less than 1 cm in diameter) with a smooth, well
defined wall and fluid contents are generally of little clinical
significance and probably represent an accumulation of
prostatic secretions. Larger cysts may cause asymmetrical
prostatic enlargement. The wall may be thick and irregular
and the centre may be septated or contain debris (Figure 7.15). Prostatic abscesses or tumours with a cystic
component may have an identical ultrasonographic appearance so needle aspiration of the contents may be required
for a definitive diagnosis (Figure 7.16).

In cases of prostatic haemorrhage, ultrasonographic
examination of the prostate is often unrewarding. Although
haematomata or haematocysts have been reported in many
instances the prostate appears ultrasonographically normal.

Diffuse parenchymal disease

Benign prostatic hypertrophy is a common condition in entire
male dogs. The prostate often appears enlarged but remains

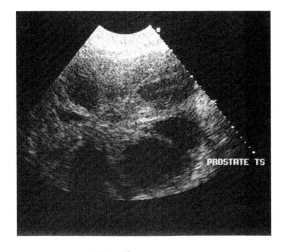

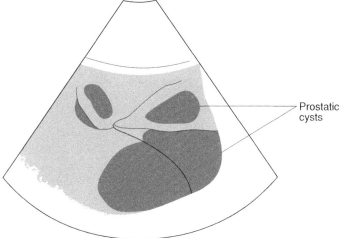

Figure 7.15   Multiple prostatic cysts in an entire dog with prostatic hyperplasia. Note the internal septations producing a cartwheel appearance. There is some solid tissue present especially around the rim.

smooth in outline and a normal shape. The echotexture is still even but a slight overall increase in echogenicity has been noted by some authors. The hilar echo is thought to become less obvious, either as a result of the overall increase in echogenicity or because of compression. In practical terms, it may be difficult to differentiate a normal prostate and a hypertrophied prostate ultrasonographically except on the basis of size. In some cases there may be single or multiple cysts throughout the prostate secondary to the hormonal change (Figure 7.17).

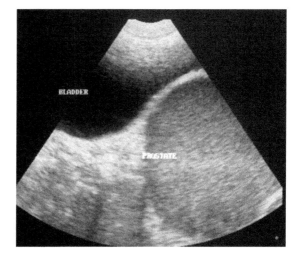

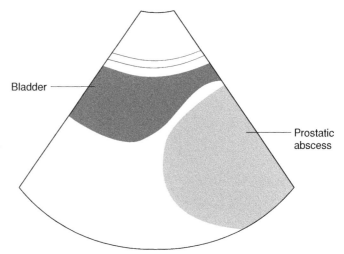

Figure 7.16 Prostatic abscess in an entire dog. The flocculent material within the abscess can be seen to be much more echogenic than the adjacent urine-filled bladder, which is quite anechoic. A thickened wall cannot be seen in this image but may be seen in some.

In acute prostatitis, the prostate is usually enlarged. In severe cases, a distinctly mottled texture is seen with an overall decrease in echogenicity. The hypoechoic patches seen presumably represent areas of haemorrhage, necrosis or abscess formation. With extension of inflammatory changes into the periprostatic tissues the outline of the prostate may become rather poorly defined.

Chronic prostatitis may also result in a patchy density but in this instance the overall impression is of an increase in echogenicity. Hyperechoic areas probably represent fibrosis

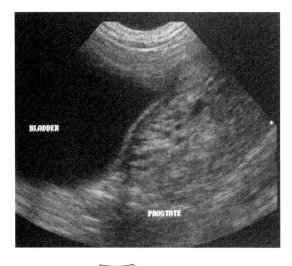

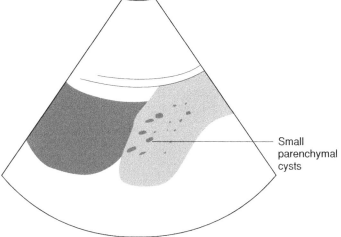

Small parenchymal cysts

Figure 7.17 Prostatic hyperplasia in an entire dog. Note the diffusely coarsened appearance produced by multiple, small parenchymal cysts.

or calcification. The gland is of variable size in such cases but may be irregular in outline.

Prostatic tumours in the dog are not usually diagnosed until they reach a relatively advanced stage. Thus localised nodules within otherwise normal prostatic parenchyma as described in man are not usually identified. Instead a moderately enlarged prostate is seen, often with irregular and indistinct margins. The echotexture is patchy with an overall increase in echogenicity. From this description it is apparent that it is difficult to differentiate prostatic neoplasia

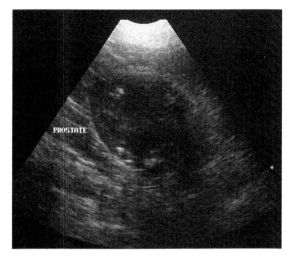

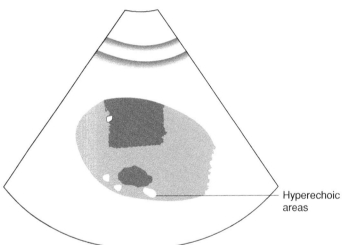

Figure 7.18 Prostatic neoplasia in an 11-year-old dog neutered at one year of age. The prostate is enlarged given the neutered status and the parenchyma is irregular with small hyperechoic areas consistent with mineralisation. Prostatomegaly in a dog neutered for some time should be considered suspicious for neoplasia.

and chronic prostatitis by ultrasonography alone. It has been suggested that focal mineralisation with acoustic shadowing is more suggestive of neoplasia than chronic prostatitis in the dog (Figure 7.18). Prostatomegaly in a neutered dog should always be considered suspicious for neoplasia and biopsies taken. The demonstration of enlarged sublumbar lymph nodes is more likely in neoplasia but may occur in cases of chronic infection. Biopsy is therefore usually required for definitive diagnosis.

Paraprostatic disease

Paraprostatic cysts vary greatly in size, shape and position. They are usually well circumscribed with thin, smooth walls and fluid contents. Internal septa are common and in some cysts the presence of multiple septa gives the appearance of a honeycomb or a sponge. A variable amount of solid tissue is present. Mineralisation of the wall of prostatic cysts is not uncommon and will be recognised ultrasonographically by the presence of acoustic shadowing. The prostate should normally be identifiable as a separate structure (Figure 7.19). It is not possible to ascertain ultrasonographically whether such cysts have a neoplastic component or not. Biopsy of the cyst wall during surgery is usually necessary to determine this.

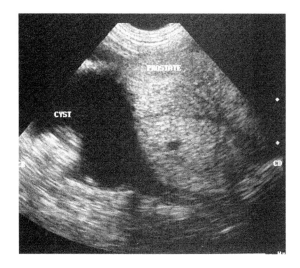

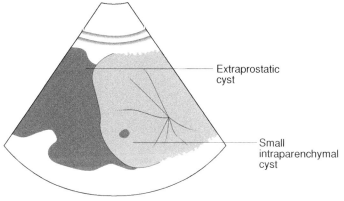

Extraprostatic cyst

Small intraparenchymal cyst

Figure 7.19
Extraprostatic/ paraprostatic cyst in an entire male dog. Note how the cyst extends cranially, separate to the bladder. A small intraparenchymal cyst can be seen within the prostate.

In cases of perineal rupture, either the bladder or the paraprostatic cyst may pass caudally into the perineum. Ultrasonography of the perineal swelling will confirm the presence of a large fluid-filled structure. If internal septa are present, the structure can be identified as a paraprostatic cyst. If the structure is smooth in outline with no divisions, it may be a simple cyst but the retroflexed urinary bladder could look similar and contrast urethrocystography will be needed to clarify the situation.

Suggested reading

Barr, F. (1990) Ultrasonographic Measurement of Normal Renal Parameters. In: *Journal of Small Animal Practice*, **31**, pp. 180–184.

Cartee, R. E. & Rowles, T. (1983) Transabdominal Sonographic Evaluation of the Canine Prostate. In: *Veterinary Radiology*, **24**, pp. 156–164.

Feeney, D. A., Johnston, G. R., Klausner, J. S., *et al.* (1987) Canine Prostatic Disease – Comparison of Ultrasonographic Appearance with Morphological and Microbiologic findings – 30 cases (1981–1985). In: *Journal of the American Veterinary Medical Association*, **190**, pp. 1027–1034.

Feeney, D. A., Johnston, G. R. & Klausner, J. S. (1985) Two-dimensional Gray-scale Ultrasonography: Application in Canine Prostatic Disease. In: *Veterinary Clinic of North America: Small Animal Practice*, **15**, pp. 1159–1176.

Nyland, T. G., Mattoon, J. S. (2002) Chapter 4: 'Abdominal Ultrasound Scanning Techniques.' In: *Small Animal Diagnostic Ultrasound*, 2nd edn, pp. 49–81. W. B. Saunders Co., Philadelphia.

Nyland, T. G., Mattoon, J. S. (2002) Chapter 9: 'Urinary Tract.' In: *Small Animal Diagnostic Ultrasound*, 2nd edn, pp. 158–195. W. B. Saunders Co., Philadelphia.

Chapter 8

Imaging of the Reproductive Tract

Alison Dickie

The uterus

Imaging procedure

The cervix in the bitch and queen is situated between the dorsal aspect of the bladder neck and the ventral aspect of the colon. Cranial to this is the short uterine body, which branches into two long uterine horns. These run cranially through the abdomen towards the ovaries, which are located caudal or caudoventral to the ipsilateral kidney.

Identification of the uterus is easiest when the ultrasound examination is performed with the animal in the standing position, as the tract maintains its normal anatomical location relative to the adjacent structures. An area of hair is clipped from the caudal ventral abdomen although this may not always be necessary since this region is often relatively hairless. If the bitch is particularly fat or has marked mammary gland development, a more lateral approach may be necessary to avoid the need for imaging at excessive depth. Patient preparation is as described elsewhere for the rest of the abdomen (see p. 26). A 7.5 MHz transducer is the most appropriate for assessment of the uterus as the depth of penetration required is relatively short and it produces high-resolution images. A 5.0 MHz transducer may also be used but image resolution will be sacrificed and the normal uterus may not be seen. Linear, microconvex, curvilinear and sector transducers are all suitable for this procedure and sedation is usually not required.

As the normal, non-gravid uterus is often difficult to locate, the bladder and colon are used as landmarks to allow visualisation of the uterus in its position between these two structures. The bladder acts as an acoustic window through which the body of the uterus can be examined and it is therefore best to perform the examination when the animal has a full bladder. The length of the tract visualised in this

145

way will depend on the degree of bladder distension. Some operators prefer to scan the uterus with the animal in lateral or dorsal recumbency, although this may result in the tract being more difficult to locate as it slips lateral to the bladder. If the uterus is enlarged either due to pregnancy or pathology, it is much easier to identify and can usually be located in the caudal abdomen without having to use the bladder as an acoustic window. Initially, short-axis images of the bladder and cervix are obtained and the long-axis views then examined.

Normal appearance

Non-gravid uterus

The transducer is placed transversely across the abdomen and the bladder is imaged in short axis. The cervix appears as a round, hypoechoic structure positioned between the anechoic bladder and the hyperechoic semi-circle representing the colon. When the transducer is moved in a cranial direction, the uterine body is imaged in short axis. It has a smaller diameter than the cervix and is relatively homogenous in appearance without an apparent lumen. Further cranial movement allows the division of the uterine body into two horns to be identified. These are oval-shaped, hypoechoic structures located one on each side of the midline (Figure 8.1). Once the transducer is advanced beyond the cranial margin of the bladder, the normal uterine horns cannot usually be easily identified within the intestinal mass. Rotation of the transducer through 90° allows the cervix and uterine body to be imaged in long axis as a hypoechoic tubular structure, narrowing cranially. The uterine horns may be difficult to image as they run off in a more lateral direction and once again, they may not be visualised beyond the cranial margin of the bladder.

The uterus is most difficult to locate in late dioestrus and anoestrus when it is less than 1 cm in diameter. Ultrasound is not, therefore, a reliable method for determining if an animal has been spayed as the uterus cannot always be imaged. Sometimes two layers are visible within the uterine walls, a central hypoechoic region representing the endometrium and an outer hyperechoic region representing the myometrium and serosa. During prooestrus and oestrus the uterus increases in diameter and becomes more homogenous in

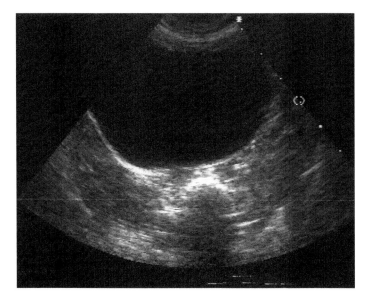

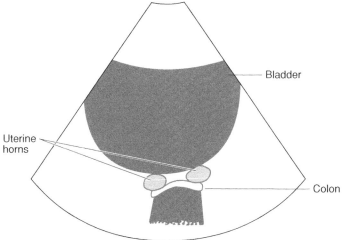

Uterine horns

Bladder

Colon

Figure 8.1 Normal uterine horns in a bitch. This is a short-axis section through the bladder and descending colon with the small, oval-shaped hypoechoic uterine horns located between them.

appearance due to the presence of oedema which results in the tract becoming much easier to identify at this stage of the cycle. This appearance is maintained into early dioestrus when the pregnant and non-pregnant tract is indistinguishable using ultrasound. At this stage of the cycle, it may be possible to image the uterine horns beyond the margins of the bladder. The uterine horns are followed through the abdomen towards the ovaries which necessitates altering the orientation of the transducer in whichever direction is required to maintain them in either long or short axis on the ultrasound image. They are easy to distinguish from loops of small intestine due to the lack of five distinct wall layers, absence of peristaltic contractions and their relatively straight course through the abdomen rather than the coiled nature of intestinal loops. The cervix is also easily identified at this stage as it is wider than the uterine body and is composed of multiple layers which appear as concentric rings on the ultrasound image when it is imaged in short axis.

Gravid uterus

Pregnancy can be identified using ultrasound as early as 17 days after the LH (luteinising hormone) surge in dogs and 11–14 days after mating in the cat. At this stage, the gestational sac is composed entirely of yolk sac and appears as a discrete, anechoic sphere within the uterine lumen measuring approximately 2 mm in diameter. Several of these sacs will be located at intervals along both uterine horns. This causes enlargement of the uterus making it much easier to identify within the abdomen without having to rely on the bladder as an acoustic window. The different layers of the uterine wall may be differentiated on the ultrasound image with the outer myometrium appearing hypoechoic and the inner endometrium relatively hyperechoic.

The embryo first becomes visible around day 21 of gestation as a small echogenic structure located close to the endometrium (Figure 8.2). Soon after this, careful examination will reveal a small flicker within the embryo representing the heartbeat and indicating viability. Some ultrasound machines have a frame-averaging function, which smoothes out the images obtained when scanning the abdomen, thus producing a picture which is more pleasing to the eye. It is important to ensure, however, that this function is switched off when trying to identify the embryonic heartbeat as the frame averaging may make it difficult to visualise this type of movement.

By day 25, the gestational sacs are approximately 1 cm in diameter and are more oval in shape than spherical. The embryo is larger, distinctly bipolar in shape and begins to move away from the endometrium making it easier to visualise (Figure 8.3). It is separated from the endometrium by an anechoic region representing the developing allantoic sac, which progressively increases in size, pushing the embryo away from the wall and into the lumen of the vesicle, as the

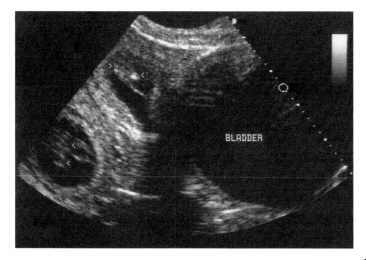

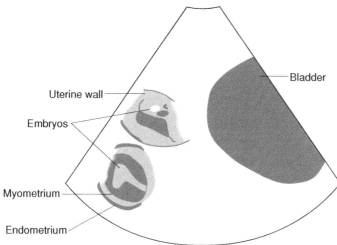

Figure 8.2 Normal pregnancy in a bitch. Two anechoic, fluid-filled gestational sacs located cranial to the bladder, each containing a small echogenic structure representing the embryo. In real-time imaging, a flickering pixel would be visible within each embryo indicating viability. The outer myometrium appears hypoechoic and the inner endometrium relatively hyperechoic.

yolk sac regresses. Eventually the allantois occupies the entire vesicle and the yolk sac remains as a folded tubular structure. Care must be taken not to mistake this for abnormal or separated fetal membranes. By day 35, the fetus has a distinct head, trunk and abdomen, and fetal movements can be observed. The developing fetal skeleton can be visualised as hyperechoic structures within the fetus and after approximately day 40, it produces increasingly marked distal acoustic shadowing as calcification progresses (Figure 8.4). Within the fetal heart, the individual chambers can be discerned and the hyperechoic heart valves can be visualised. Other anatomical features such as the fluid-filled fetal

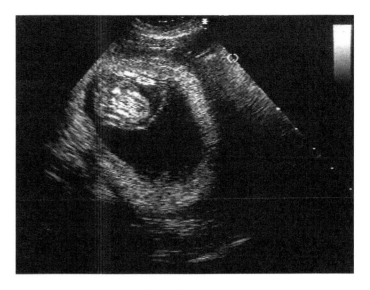

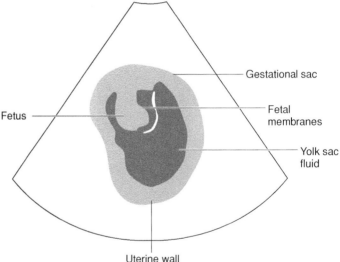

Figure 8.3 Normal 26 day pregnancy in a bitch. The oval-shaped gestational sac contains an echogenic embryo, which is separated from the uterine wall by the developing anechoic allantois.

stomach, urinary bladder and great vessels can be identified as anechoic structures. The lungs are not yet air filled and so appear as an echogenic region within the fetal rib cage surrounding the heart. The lungs are hyperechoic relative to the liver and so a distinct line representing the position of the diaphragm can also be identified. Towards the end of pregnancy, the fetal kidneys and intestines become visible. The placenta in the bitch and queen is zonary and forms a band around the centre of the conceptus, which is sometimes visualised as a localised, sausage-shaped thickening

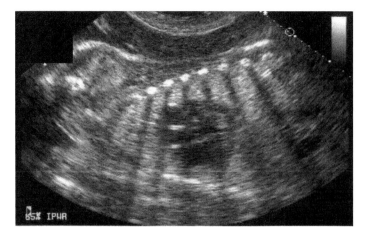

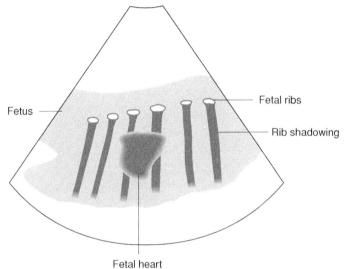

Fetus

Fetal ribs

Rib shadowing

Fetal heart

Figure 8.4 Normal pregnancy greater than day 42 in a bitch. The mineralised fetal ribs appear hyperechoic and produce distal acoustic shadowing. The anechoic heart is visible in the centre of the thorax surrounded by echogenic lung tissue.

of the endometrium in this region (Figure 8.5). The fetus remains mobile within the membranes so its location relative to this structure is variable.

Although ultrasound allows identification of the conceptus very early in gestation, when performing routine pregnancy diagnosis in the bitch it is advisable to wait until at least 28 days following the last mating. This is due to the variable time interval between mating and conception in dogs and will reduce the chances of a false negative result. The embryonic vesicles are large enough to identify and the embryonic heartbeats will be sufficiently visible to confirm viability even if the bitch has had a 'late mating' and the concepti are younger than than anticipated. Scanning prior to 28 days may also

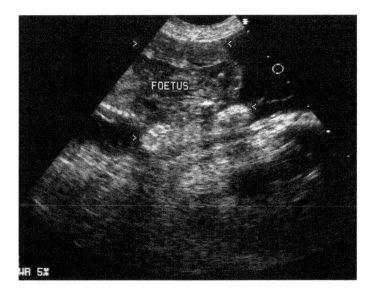

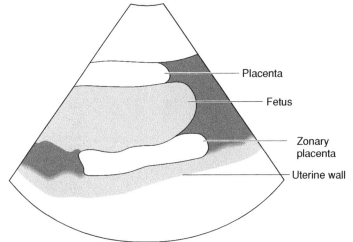

Figure 8.5 Normal placenta in a bitch. The sausage-shaped echogenic structure of the zonary placenta is visible around the fetus, which remains mobile within the allantoic sac.

result in false positive diagnoses if uterine cysts or other small fluid-filled structures within the abdomen are misidentified as embryonic vesicles. Also, since the embryo is not visible, viability cannot be assessed. The cat is an induced ovulator and so there is better correlation between the time of mating and the stage of gestation in this species. An accurate diagnosis can be achieved around 20–21 days after mating when the embryo will be visible.

An approximation of gestational age can be obtained by measuring various parameters associated with the concepti. The most appropriate measurement will be dictated by the stage of gestation and the position of the fetuses which will affect the images obtained. Early in gestation, the diameter of each vesicle can be measured easily until they become too large to be contained within the screen of the ultrasound machine. Following this, the crown–rump length of a fetus can be measured by obtaining a long-axis view. This is easy to perform until each fetus itself becomes too large and only sections of it can be imaged on the screen at any one time. At this stage the trunk diameter, which is measured across the diameter of the abdomen at the level of the um-bilical cord, or the biparietal diameter, measured across the width of the skull can be used, depending on which views are obtained of the fetus (Figure 8.6). Many veterinary

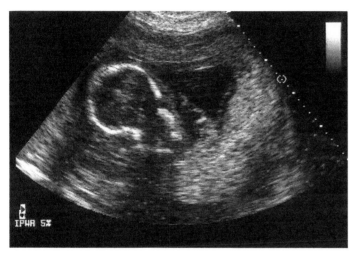

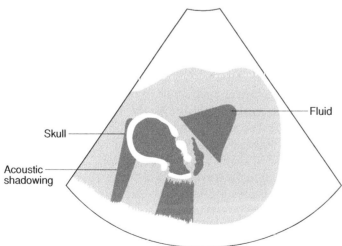

Figure 8.6 Normal canine fetus. Short-axis view across the skull of a fetus, which would be suitable for the performance of a bi-parietal measurement to calculate gestational age. The hyperechoic, mineralised bones of the skull are producing distal acoustic shadowing.

ultrasound machines now incorporate gestational age calculation packages where the machine will estimate the gestational age of the fetus to within a range of approximately
five days from a specific measurement. Alternatively, the
stage of organ development can be assessed and compared
to published tables. The progression of pregnancy in the cat
is very similar to that of the dog.

It is not advisable to attempt to accurately determine the
litter size using ultrasound, as this is notoriously problematic,
especially later in gestation when the fetuses are large and
overlie one another. As they cannot be imaged individually or
on a single slice it is very difficult to ensure that a conceptus
has not been either missed or counted twice. Determining
numbers is more accurate when performed between approximately 27 and 37 days of gestation when each conceptus
is large enough to be identified easily but is still a discrete
structure. Accuracy is improved in smaller litters while large
ones are usually underestimated. It is therefore probably
safer to limit the prediction to greater than or less than five.

Post-partum uterus

Ultrasound can also be used to examine the post-partum
uterus in the bitch. This is larger in diameter than the normal
non-pregnant tract, resulting in uterine horns which can
easily be followed beyond the cranial margin of the bladder
and through the intestines towards the ovaries. The lumen
contains varying amounts of anechoic or echogenic fluid
depending on the amount of blood or placental debris remaining. The endometrium appears as a distinct but irregular
hyperechoic layer although its internal margin may not
be clearly visualised if the luminal material is of a similar
echogenicity or if the adjacent lumen is empty, resulting in
apposition of the endometrial surfaces. The myometrium is
a distinct but irregular hypoechoic layer and the outer serosal
layer appears hyperechoic due to the presence of fat and
fibrous tissue between it and the myometrium. Placental
sites can be identified as thicker regions throughout the uterus
and are ovoid in shape when imaged in long axis. Immediately post partum, the uterus has a diameter of approximately
2.5 cm at the placental sites and 1.25 cm at the intervening
regions.

The diameter of the uterus will reduce with time as
involution progresses and the luminal contents increase in

echogenicity, due to the expulsion of the remaining fluid, leaving cellular material and debris. Despite reaching a similar diameter, it is still easy to differentiate the involuting uterus from loops of small intestine on the basis of the number of wall layers present and an absence of peristalsis. In addition, although there is an increase in the echogenicity of the uterine luminal contents, they are still not as echogenic as the intestinal contents and there should be no acoustic shadowing due to the absence of gas. However, as the diameter decreases, it may become difficult to image the entire uterus due to interference from intestinal gas, although it should still be possible to image the body at least up to approximately six weeks post partum when the placental sites can still be identified sonographically. The uterus returns to a normal diameter around four to six weeks post partum, although it does not appear sonographically normal until approximately 15 weeks post partum.

Uterine involution occurs much more rapidly in the queen with the uterine diameter decreasing to less than 1 cm after 14 days post partum and being considered as sonographically complete by 24 days. Despite similar zonary placentation, it is not possible to identify placental sites, although this may be due to the smaller overall size of the uterus in the queen relative to the bitch. This may also be responsible for a failure to differentiate distinct wall layers in all cases although these should be imaged up until day 14. Otherwise, ultrasound imaging of uterine involution in the queen is similar to that of the bitch.

Abnormal appearance

Ultrasound is a rapid and non-invasive method for monitoring pregnancies and also assessing fetal well-being throughout gestation. Indications of a distressed fetus include a reduction in fetal movement and a slowing of the heart rate to less than twice that of the mother. (The fetal heart rate can be determined using M mode.) Loss of the fetal heartbeat is the most reliable indication of fetal death. Subsequently there is resorption of the fetal fluids, the remaining fluid becomes echogenic and the fetus becomes less distinct on the ultrasound image as it begins to degenerate. Spontaneous resorption of concepti is relatively common early in gestation and the rest of the pregnancy may continue normally. However, in the third trimester of pregnancy, abortion of the entire litter is more likely to be the result. Following abortion of fetuses the appearance of the uterus is similar to that of the post-partum uterus.

Ultrasound can also be used to assess fetal well-being approaching or during parturition as the identification of stressed or dead fetuses will have an influence on how the case is managed. In addition, the detection of retained fetuses is possible if parturition has become interrupted or ceased. When checking for retained fetuses, it is important to scan right up into the pelvic cavity as often a fetus will be located in the cervical or vaginal portion of the tract and could be easily missed.

Abnormalities of the post-partum uterus include fetal or placental retention, haemorrhage following trauma to the uterus at parturition, subinvolution of placental sites and post-partum endometritis. However, it may be difficult to differentiate between the retention of placental material or the presence of pus or haemorrhage and the normal debris which is retained for a variable length of time within the uterus following parturition. The most reliable indicator of normal involution is therefore a return to a normal diameter and failure to do so is likely to be associated with one of the conditions previously mentioned.

Pyometra is a common condition, particularly in older entire bitches, and ultrasound provides a rapid, safe and non-invasive method of diagnosis. A closed pyometra is easily identified by the presence of distended, fluid-filled loops of uterine horn which can occupy a large area of the abdominal cavity and are readily visualised if the transducer is placed anywhere on the ventral abdominal wall (Figure 8.7). The thickness of the uterine wall can be variable depending on the degree of distension and the luminal contents may be anechoic or contain echogenic material depending on their composition. The distended uterine horns can easily be followed cranially beyond the margin of the bladder and identified within the intestinal mass. They can be readily differentiated from loops of small intestine as previously described (see p. 148). In addition, it is possible to follow the tubular structure caudally to a region between the colon and bladder representing the body of the uterus and cranially towards the kidneys.

Ultrasound is very sensitive for identifying even small accumulations of fluid within the uterine lumen in the early stages of this condition (Figure 8.8). In these cases, the

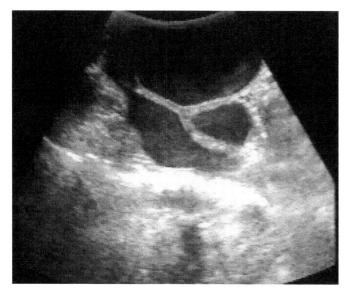

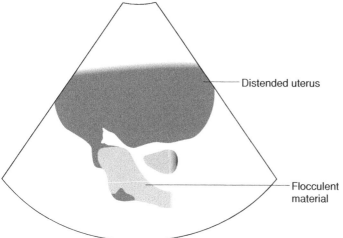

Distended uterus

Flocculent
material

Figure 8.7 Closed
pyometra in a cat. The
large, distended, fluid-
filled loops of uterine
horn are easily
visualised within the
caudal abdomen and
contain flocculent
echogenic material
representing cellular
debris.

intraluminal fluid is best identified in the caudal area of the
uterine horns and the uterine body using the bladder as an
acoustic window. Pyometra also occurs in the queen and
can follow spontaneous or mating-induced ovulations. The
findings are similar to those observed in the bitch.

Identification of an open pyometra may be more difficult
due to constant drainage through the open cervix, preventing
the accumulation of enough fluid to produce any appreciable
distension of the uterine lumen on ultrasound examination.
Increasing the frequency of the transducer may help to

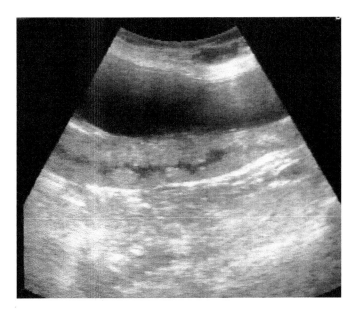

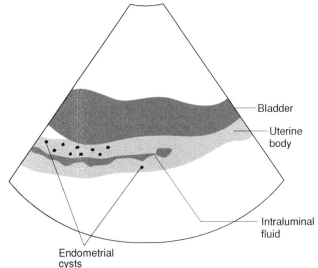

Figure 8.8 Pyometra and cystic endometrial hyperplasia in a bitch. A small volume of intraluminal uterine fluid, in association with multiple, small, anechoic cysts located throughout the endometrium, indicates the presence of cystic endometrial hyperplasia.

Bladder

Uterine body

Intraluminal fluid

Endometrial cysts

visualise these small volumes but this is still not always possible and so the presence of an open pyometra cannot be ruled out on the basis of an apparently normal sonographic appearance of the uterus.

Cystic endometrial hyperplasia occurs during the luteal phase of the oestrous cycle as a result of the influence of progesterone and causes multiple anechoic cysts of varying diameter which are scattered throughout the uterus. They may be poorly defined and are asymmetrical in position as they are embedded within the endometrium rather than being located in the uterine lumen. A small volume of free luminal fluid may also be identified and it has been suggested that cystic endometrial hyperplasia may be a precursor to pyometra (Figure 8.8). Some cases may be difficult to identify using ultrasound if the gross changes are too subtle or the cysts too small for detection. However, increasing the frequency of the transducer may allow more subtle changes to be identified. An exaggerated form of cystic endometrial hyperplasia may occasionally be observed in the presence of an active ovarian tumour with a series of large cysts developing throughout the entire uterus. Care must be taken to differentiate these from embryonic vesicles by ascertaining the absence of an embryo with a visible heart beat, echogenic rather than anechoic contents and a failure to increase in size over time and develop at a rate consistent with an embryonic vesicle. Uterine tumours are uncommon and have a very variable sonographic appearance.

Abnormalities of the uterine stump may be identified in spayed bitches exhibiting a persistent vaginal discharge or dysuria and are most commonly due to post-operative infection. These stump pyometras, granulomas or abscesses can have a very variable appearance on ultrasound with irregular margins and mixed echogenicity but the anatomical location between the bladder neck and descending colon confirms the tissue of origin (Figure 8.9). Tumours can also arise from the region of the uterine stump and these also have a variable sonographic appearance. The only way to differentiate these conditions is by taking a fine-needle aspirate or biopsy of the region, both of which can be performed under ultrasound guidance. If a lesion is identified in the region of the uterine stump or bladder neck, it is important to check the kidneys, as obstruction of the distal ureters will result in secondary hydronephrosis and this will have an influence on how the case is managed.

The ovary

Imaging procedure

The ovaries are small structures and can be difficult to image depending on the stage of the oestrous cycle and also the body condition of the animal. A high frequency transducer, such as 7.5 MHz, is required in order to adequately visualise

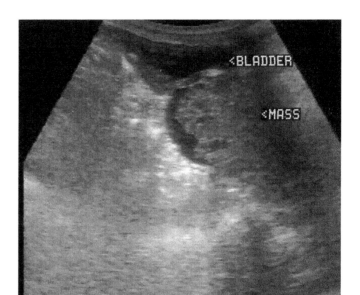

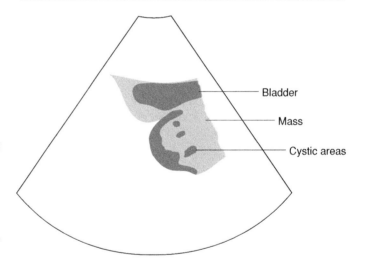

Figure 8.9 Stump pyometra in a bitch. Large mass of mixed echogenicity containing several irregularly shaped cystic areas located between the bladder and the descending colon, indicating that it is arising from the uterine stump.

the various structures within the ovary and this is possible due to the relatively superficial position of the ovary. The ovary in the cat may require a 10–15 MHz transducer for identification.

It is possible to examine the ovaries with the animal in lateral recumbency or in a standing position, although the former may be preferable in order to reduce movement of the patient. However, the exact location of the ovaries within the abdomen will vary depending on the position of the animal and this should be borne in mind when trying to locate them. An area of hair is clipped in the sublumbar region caudal to the last rib on both flanks and the caudal pole of the kidney is identified as a landmark. In lateral recumbency, the ovary is in the region caudal to the ipsilateral kidney but in the standing position it will move to a more ventral and lateral position under gravity. It is not usually possible to visualise the ovaries from the ventral abdominal wall due to the presence of intervening gas-filled intestine.

Normal appearance

The ease of location and sonographic appearance of the ovaries depends on the structures present within them and therefore the stage of oestrous cycle. Anoestrous ovaries do not contain any distinct structures and are small, oval-shaped, homogenous structures, which are hypoechoic relative to the surrounding tissue. They can therefore easily be overlooked especially if the animal is fat, and consequently failure to identify ovaries using ultrasound is not a reliable method of determining whether the animal has been spayed.

The presence of active structures such as follicles and corpora lutea increases the size of the ovaries therefore making them easier to identify during oestrous and dioestrous. The appearance of individual structures will depend on the quality of the equipment used but follicles generally appear as round, fluid-filled, anechoic areas, while corpora lutea are homogenous echogenic structures which may have a hypoechoic or anechoic centre (Figure 8.10). However, pre-ovulatory follicles and early corpora lutea can have a very similar sonographic appearance and so ultrasound is not a reliable method for detecting the occurrence of ovulation unless serial examinations are performed and this is extremely time consuming. The developing follicles do not project beyond the margins of the ovary so it maintains its smoothly marginated oval shape until around the time of ovulation, after which the developing corpora lutea, which do protrude beyond the margins, produce a more irregular and knobbly outline to the ovary.

Abnormal appearance

Ovarian masses

Ultrasound is useful for the identification and investigation of ovarian masses, however these are uncommon in the

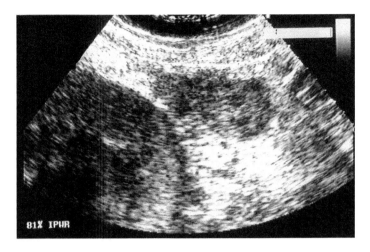

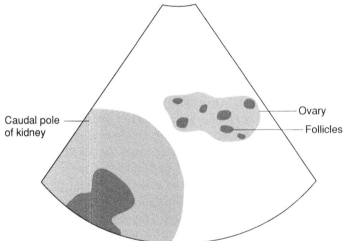

Caudal pole of kidney

Ovary

Follicles

Figure 8.10 Normal ovary in a bitch. It is located adjacent to the caudal pole of the ipsilateral kidney and contains several fluid-filled follicles.

bitch due to the high incidence of spaying. The most common types are papillary and granulosa cell tumours, although there are a wide range of types possible and they can be unilateral or bilateral. The affected ovary is enlarged and is identified by its location caudal to the respective kidney. As the ovary enlarges it moves ventrally within the abdomen due to stretching of the mesovarium and it therefore becomes more difficult to distinguish from tumours arising from other abdominal organs.

Ovarian tumours

Ovarian tumours can demonstrate a wide range of sonographic appearances. However, they commonly have a solid hypoechoic component in association with either single or multiple anechoic cystic areas, although some may be entirely cystic in nature. The presence of solid material increases the chances of the lesions being malignant and the anechoic areas may represent regions of necrosis and hae-morrhage. Most ovarian tumours have well defined margins which can vary from smooth through irregular to nodular in outline. Granulosa cell tumours may produce a charac-teristic honeycomb pattern on ultrasound and theoretically, teratomas containing teeth should produce a hyperechoic image with distal acoustic shadowing, although this is not commonly observed. It is not possible to determine the tumour type on the basis of the ultrasound images alone.

Ovarian tumours may be imaged in association with free abdominal fluid but it is not usually possible to actually visualise the presence of abdominal metastases. Abnormal-ities of the uterus, including pyometra and cystic endometrial hyperplasia, are also often identified in association with ovarian tumours although it is not clear whether these are related or coincidental findings.

Ovarian cysts

Ovarian cysts are a common abnormality of the canine ovary and appear as discrete, oval-shaped, anechoic structures with thin walls. This may result in an appearance similar to that of a normal oestrous or early dioestrous ovary at an inap-propriate stage of the cycle. Multiple cysts within an ovary may appear either as a cluster of individual anechoic struc-tures or as a single, larger, irregular-shaped structure de-pending on whether the walls separating the cysts are well visualised or not. Individual cysts can enlarge up to around 20 cm in diameter. In these cases, it is important to rule out the possibility of the cystic structure being within another abdominal organ before the diagnosis of an ovarian cyst can be reached. Most ovarian cysts are benign but if a multi-cystic ovary is imaged, which also contains a large amount of echogenic tissue, then the possibility of an ovarian tumour should also be considered.

An inability to identify ovaries on ultrasound does not allow their absence to be confirmed. Likewise, the identi-fication of ovarian remnants following spaying is difficult unless the tissue contains prominent structures such as follicles or cysts.

The testes

Imaging procedure

Clipping is not usually required when performing an ultrasound examination of the canine testes as, in most cases, the skin surface of the scrotum is relatively hairless. It is most convenient to examine the testes with the dog in lateral recumbency to reduce movement of the patient, although if the operator prefers, it can also be performed with the dog standing. Depending on the type of transducer used, there may be some loss of image quality associated with the area of the testicle nearest to the transducer as a result of near-field distortion due to close apposition of the testicle to the transducer face. This is most commonly encountered when using sector or microconvex transducers due to the shape of the beam. It can be prevented either by placing a sonolucent stand-off pad between the transducer and the skin surface, or by imaging one testicle through the other using the one nearest to the transducer as a natural anatomical stand-off to increase the distance between the scan face and the area of interest. This is particularly useful when imaging a small or atrophied testicle. A high frequency transducer such as 7.5 MHz or higher is ideal for imaging the testicle as the depth of penetration required is small and the resolution of the resulting image is good. Each testicle should be imaged from a variety of different angles including sagittal, transverse and dorsal planes to ensure that the entire organ has been examined.

Ultrasound examination of the testes of the cat is not commonly indicated and so will not be discussed further. However, the sonographic appearance will be similar to that of the dog, although clipping of the adjacent perineal region will be required.

Normal appearance

The parenchyma of each testicle is coarse and granular with a homogenous medium echogenicity similar to that of the spleen or prostate. The connective tissue mediastinum testes appears as a hyperechoic line in the centre of the testicle when it is imaged in long axis and a dot when imaged in short axis and is approximately 2 mm in diameter (Figure 8.11). Occasionally, hyperechoic flecks are visualised within the parenchyma which represents radiating sheets of connective tissue

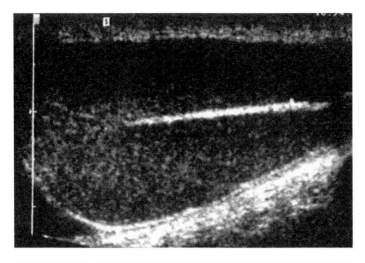

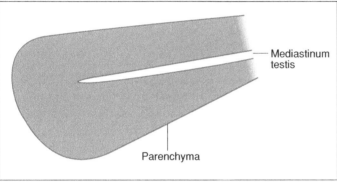

Mediastinum
testis

Parenchyma

Figure 8.11 Normal
testicle in a dog.
Long-axis view
demonstrating the
coarse, evenly
echogenic parenchyma
and the hyperechoic
linear structure of the
mediastinum testes.

from the mediastinum extending between the parenchymal
sections. The dimensions of both testes are usually similar.

The tail of the epididymis is located at the caudal pole of
the testicle and is easy to identify as a coiled hypoechoic
structure. The head is located at the cranial pole and the body
runs along the dorsomedial aspect of the testicle although
it is less consistently imaged. The fibrous tunics are visible
around the periphery of the testes as a hyperechoic capsule and
there should be no peritesticular fluid identified in the dog.

Abnormal appearance

Testicular masses

Ultrasound is useful in investigating testicular masses and
there are several types of testicular neoplasia which occur in
the dog, although their appearance is very variable on ultrasound. Seminomas or Sertoli-cell tumours are more likely

to be large with a mixed echogenicity and may extend to involve the entire testicle producing marked disruption of the normal architecture. Interstitial cell adenomas may produce more focal, well defined, solid hypoechoic mass lesions. However, in all cases, areas of haemorrhage and necrosis may occur producing disorganised hypoechoic areas. Ultrasound is therefore not diagnostic for tumour type although it will identify lesions situated within the substance of the testicle which cannot be palpated (Figure 8.12).

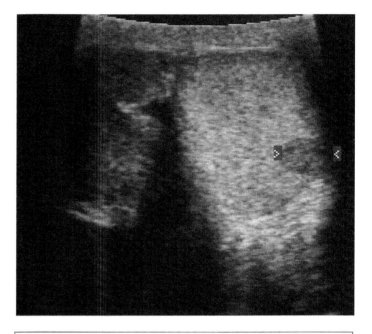

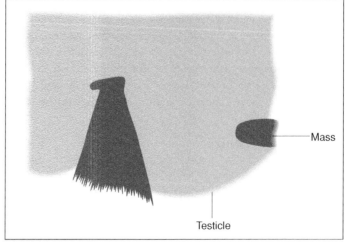

Figure 8.12
Interstitial cell adenoma in a dog. The mass is visible as a small, hypoechoic nodule within the otherwise apparently normal parenchyma of the testicle.

Areas of calcification within the testicle appear as hyper-echoic foci producing distal acoustic shadowing and may be associated with neoplasia or identified as an incidental finding in an otherwise apparently normal testicle. Testicular atrophy is characterised by the presence of a small, hypoechoic, homogenous testicle while orchitis results in a large, painful testicle with a patchy appearance and hypoechoic regions throughout (Figure 8.13).

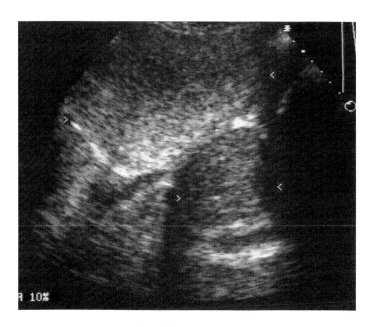

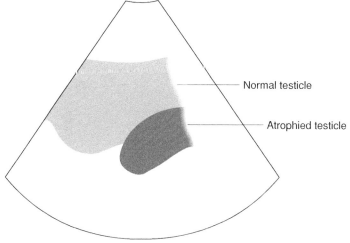

Normal testicle

Atrophied testicle

Figure 8.13
Testicular atrophy in a dog. The small, atrophied testicle is imaged using the contralateral normal one as a natural anatomical stand-off.

Peri-testicular problems

Ultrasound can be used to distinguish between abnormalities within and outside the testicle. Inflammation or oedema within the walls of the scrotum may result in an increased thickness of the layers around the testicle. The accumulation of peri-testicular fluid appears as an anechoic region between the hyperechoic tunic of the testicle and the scrotal

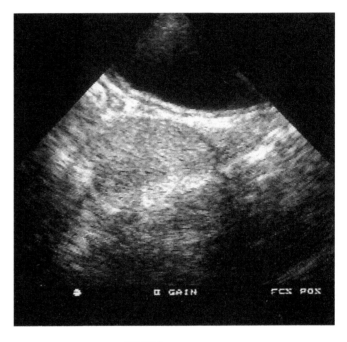

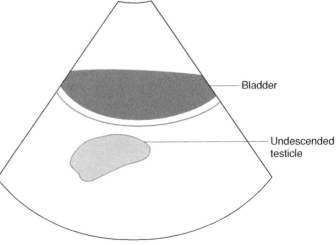

Figure 8.14
Undescended intra-abdominal testicle in a dog. It is identified as a homogeneous mass located cranial to the urinary bladder.

wall, the size of which will vary with the volume of fluid. This can be observed in association with a variety of conditions and the echogenicity will vary depending on the contents of the fluid and the underlying cause. It is also possible to identify the presence of a scrotal hernia when fat and small intestinal loops may be identified within the scrotum.

Retained testicle

A sonographic examination is occasionally requested in an attempt to locate a retained, intra-abdominal testicle. However, these structures are usually small and hypoplastic, which makes their identification by this method difficult. The examination should commence in the inguinal region before moving cranially to the area surrounding the bladder and bladder neck. Occasionally they may be located just cranial to the bladder (Figure 8.14). The area between the caudal pole of the ipsilateral kidney and the cranial aspect of the bladder should then be examined, although interference from gas within the intestine is often a problem. Retained testicles, which have undergone neoplastic transformation, are easier to locate due to their increased size and abnormal architecture. They appear as masses of mixed echogenicity and varying diameter, which are located in the regions of the abdomen as described above. However, it is necessary to confirm that the mass is not arising from another abdominal organ before this diagnosis can be reached.

Suggested reading

Beck, K. A., Baldwin, C. J. & Bosu, W. T. K. (1990) Ultrasound Prediction of Parturition in Queens. In: *Veterinary Radiology*, **31**, pp. 32–35.

Diez-Bru, N., Garcia-Real, I., Martinez, E. M., *et al.* (1998) Ultrasonographic Appearance of Ovarian Tumours in 10 Dogs. In: *Veterinary Radiology and Ultrasound*, **39**, pp. 226–233.

Ferretti, L. M., Newell, S. M., Graham, J. P. & Roberts, G. D. (2000) Radiography and Ultrasonography of the Normal Feline Post-partum Uterus. In: *Veterinary Radiology and Ultrasound*, **41**, pp. 287–291.

Pharr, J. W. & Post, K. (1992) Ultrasonography and Radiography of the Canine Post-partum Uterus. In: *Veterinary Radiology and Ultrasound*, **33**, pp. 35–40.

Pugh, C. R. & Konde, L. J. (1991) Sonographic Evaluation of Canine Testicular and Scrotal Abnormalities: A Review of 26 Cases. In: *Veterinary Radiology and Ultrasound*, **32**, pp. 243–250.

Pugh, C. R., Konde, L. J. & Park, R. D. (1990) Testicular Ultrasonography in the Normal Dog. In: *Veterinary Radiology and Ultrasound*, **31**, pp. 195–199.

Chapter 9

Non-Cardiac Thoracic Ultrasound

Paddy Mannion

Imaging technique

Ultrasound examination of the thoracic cavity is hampered by the surrounding bony rib cage and the air-filled lungs within. However, where an acoustic window can be obtained, this is an increasingly widely used technique for assessment of pleural, pulmonary and mediastinal disease, and assessment of the diaphragm. Perhaps one of the most significant advantages of ultrasound is that fluid and soft tissue may be distinguished, so that effusions secondary to an intrathoracic mass or diaphragmatic rupture can be distinguished from those of primary origin. This is useful for effective case management.

In general, little patient preparation is required prior to non-cardiac thoracic ultrasound, although if the patient is to be sedated or anaesthetised it is preferable that they have been starved in advance. In cases where there is respiratory distress, pre-oxygenation of the patient is very helpful as this increases the safety of the procedure. Patients with respiratory distress must be regarded as high-risk cases. If a patient is severely distressed it may be possible to provide oxygen throughout the procedure using a sealed Elizabethan collar through which oxygen is introduced. This again may increase the safety of the procedure but may not be well tolerated by some. It is often preferable for the patient to be sedated and there is a variety of agents available. In general, the combination of a sedative and analgesic is most appropriate, but this should be tailored for the individual situation. Where biopsy is considered it is essential that some form of chemical restraint with analgesia be used as the introduction of a needle through the intrathoracic muscles is painful and it is essential that the needle tip be kept in sight throughout.

Ultrasound examination is preceded by radiography with orthogonal projections of the thoracic cavity being preferred. This is essential to allow accurate positioning of the lesion and therefore permit the correct ultrasound approach. In those cases where a pleural effusion or disrupted diaphragm is suspected from the signalment and clinical examination, it is fully justified to proceed straight to ultrasound and perhaps radiograph later when the patient has been made comfortable. Ultrasound examination is only possible through an acoustic window and scan approaches may include parasternal, suprasternal (through the thoracic inlet), subcostal (through the liver) or directly over the lesion. Parasternal and lesion directed are perhaps the most commonly employed. Suprasternal is useful for assessment of the cranial mediastinum in some cases. The subcostal approach is especially useful for lesions in the caudal lung lobes and the caudal mediastinum. For small dogs and cats, a 7.5 MHz transducer is appropriate and this applies for the cranial mediastinum and the more superficial lesions even in larger dogs. However, for deeper lesions in the larger breeds, a 5 MHz transducer is required. It is useful to remember that the higher frequency produces superior resolution but allows a shallower area of examination, such that a 10 MHz transducer is useful up to approximately 4 cm, 7.5 MHz is useful up to approximately 6 cm depth, and a 5 MHz up to 15 cm depth. Because of the bony ribcage, a sector or a microconvex transducer is required to allow penetration between the ribs.

The standard sonographic approach is parasternal and this is initially used unless contra-indicated. The patient is placed in lateral recumbency with the affected side uppermost. The examination is directed immediately over the area of interest. In some cases, especially where the lesion is small and surrounded by air-filled lung, it is preferable to have the area of interest dependent so that surrounding lung tissue is collapsed and visualisation is improved. This is also the case where there is a small volume of free pleural fluid, which helps provide an acoustic window. It is however easier to biopsy with the affected side uppermost. The mid mediastinal area is evaluated by locating the heart and then scanning adjacent to this. The cranial mediastinum is evaluated by scanning cranial to this, directly under the arm and towards the point of the sternum. The most cranial region of the mediastinum is imaged from the supracostal approach and the transducer is introduced at the thoracic inlet. This is only useful in a limited number of cases. The caudal mediastinum is only really seen through the liver unless there is free pleural fluid, which will provide an acoustic window.

Where there is respiratory distress the patient is maintained in sternal recumbency or standing and the scan directed towards the affected area. This may make it more difficult to evaluate the cranial mediastinum fully but increases patient safety markedly.

Normal appearance

The normal appearance must be familiar before the abnormal can be reliably and safely detected and deciphered. Due to reflection of 99% of the sound beam at the interface of the lung and soft tissue, it is not possible to image beyond the most superficial layer of normal lung tissue. Therefore, when the transducer is applied to the intercostal spaces, with the exception of the acoustic window afforded by the heart, typical reverberation artefact is seen. The heart is generally seen from both the right and left sides roughly between rib spaces 3 to 7. This is subject to slight individual variation and so, the apex beat is often used to indicate the most appropriate site.

The cranial mediastinal vessels may be seen in a cranial location and these appear tubular when viewed in longitudinal section and round when viewed in transverse section. These are more reliably identified using both pulsed-wave and colour-flow Doppler, if these modalities are available. Caution should be exercised while taking biopsies of this area if it is not possible to define the blood vessels. Their course is quite straight though they do branch. This is important, as in many cases their course is deviated if a mediastinal mass is present (Figure 9.1).

Abnormal appearance

Pleural effusion

The sonographic appearance of a pleural effusion varies with the character and volume of fluid present. Fluids such as transudate and modified transudate are usually totally black with the pleural reflections seen as fine echogenic lines 'floating' in the surrounding fluid (Figure 9.2). As the cellular content of the fluid increases it becomes more echogenic and may even, in some cases, develop an almost granular appearance. Occasionally, if the fluid is localised, it may be possible to confuse this with a hypoechoic mass.

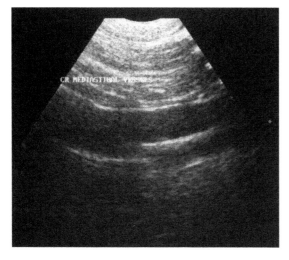

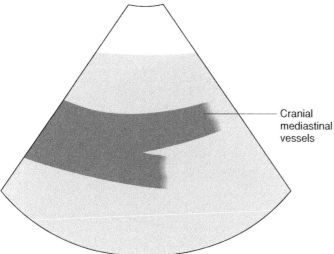

Cranial
mediastinal
vessels

Figure 9.1 Cranial mediastinal vessels. This longitudinal scan of the normal cranial mediastinum shows the branching mediastinal vessels. When viewed in transverse section these are round. Both colour-flow and pulsed-wave Doppler, may be helpful in differentiating rounded anechoic masses from blood vessels.

When fluid is an exudate or haemorrhage there may be surrounding inflammation so that the pleural surfaces become thickened and irregular. This is seen on the pleural reflections and around the pericardium and may be found with pyothorax, e.g. *Nocardia spp.*, and in some cases of long-standing chylothorax or haemorrhage (Figure 9.3). By scanning forward into the mediastinal area the pleural fluid may be seen in some cases within two separate sacs extending on either side of the mediastinum, which contains the characteristic mediastinal vessels (Figure 9.2).

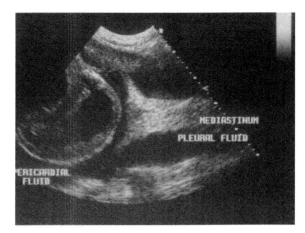

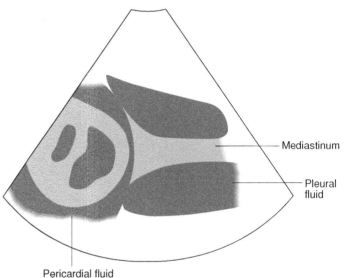

Figure 9.2 Anechoic pleural effusion. In this cat with heart disease the anechoic effusion seen within both pleural sacs and highlighting the more echogenic mediastinum, is a transudate. Note the clean and clear appearance of the pleural surfaces and notice also the moderate pericardial effusion seen in some cases.

Mediastinal masses

Masses contained within the cranial and middle mediastinum are most easily seen, although occasionally caudal mediastinal masses may be visualised. This is generally only possible if the liver or surrounding pleural fluid is used to provide an acoustic window. It is important to realise that there is no single appearance which may be attributed to a particular disease process. However, it is important to assess the margination of the mass, its relationship to the mediastinal

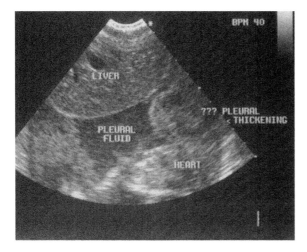

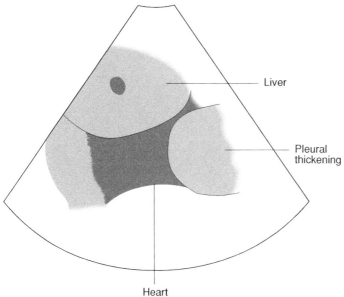

Liver

Pleural thickening

Heart

Figure 9.3 Echogenic pleural effusion. In this dog with *Nocardia* infection there is notable thickening of the pleural surfaces suggesting inflammation, while the modest volume of fluid seen is quite echogenic due to its high cell content. The amount of fluid seen on the ultrasound examination is often much less than thoracic radiographs suggest. This ultrasound appearance is typical for this type of infection.

vessels and its echogenicity. It is also important to determine if this is single or whether there are in fact multiple masses present. In some cases this can be difficult where a mass is large and lobulated. In general, neoplastic conditions are likely to have well defined borders while inflammatory conditions are more irregular and nebulous. Pulsed-wave and colour-flow Doppler examination of the mediastinum is helpful, identifying the mediastinal vessels and assessing the vascularity of the mass itself. This may be important for surgical planning.

Lymphoma

The typical appearance of lymphoma is of rounded, discrete, hypoechoic masses. These often have a fine echogenic capsule and a central echogenic line (Figure 9.4). However, a variety of other appearances may be found. In some cases the mass may be of mixed echogenicity so that areas that are hypoechoic, hyperechoic and of moderate echogenicity

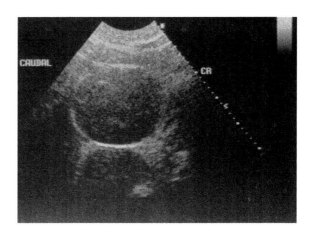

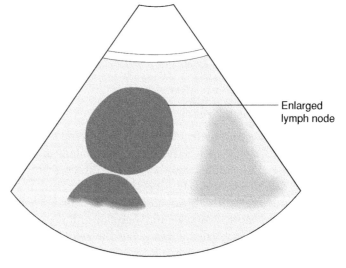

Figure 9.4 Typical appearance of lymphoma. In this young Golden Retreiver the 'typical' appearance of lymphoma in the cranial mediastinal lymph nodes can be seen. The node is rounded and hypoechoic with a smooth hyperechoic capsule. There may be a fine hyperechoic line centrally. Notice also the mirror-image artefact distant to the node itself. It is important to remember that this is only one of the many appearances seen with lymphoma.

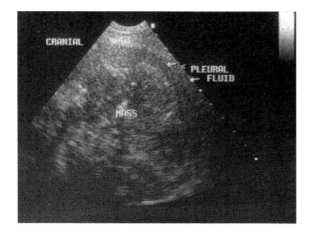

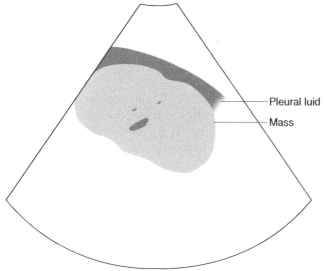

Pleural luid

Mass

Figure 9.5 Mass of mixed echogenicity. In this dog with a cranial mediastinal mass there is a small amount of surrounding fluid which is barely distinguishable from the mass itself. The edges of the mass can be seen but it has a mixed echogenicity throughout.

are intermixed (Figure 9.5). These are perhaps more likely to be larger masses. In rare cases the mass may actually appear cystic. The positioning adjacent to the mediastinal vessels is characteristic and regardless of echogenicity they are usually quite discrete. This is a useful differentiation between neoplasia and inflammation, where the latter tends to be less clearly defined in nature. The position of the vessels is very important, as this will determine whether or not surgical debulking is possible. While the discrete hypo-echoic mass with a hyperechoic rim is almost pathognomonic for lymphoma, the other appearances cannot be differentiated on the ultrasound appearance from, for example, thymoma or undifferentiated sarcoma.

Thymoma

Thymomas are mediastinal masses arising from the remnants of the thymus. They may occur in any age of animal and have a variety of appearances. They are usually cranial mediastinal in origin but if large enough may extend into the middle mediastinum also. They are well marginated but may be irregular or smooth in outline. Usually they have a moderate echogenicity but in many cases there is a mixed appearance.

Thymoma cannot be differentiated from lymphoma unless biopsies are taken. Needle-aspirate biopsies may be less rewarding than a larger sample, although in many cases they will allow a diagnosis to be made.

Mediastinitis

Inflammation of the mediastinum may have a variety of appearances and is given a separate category. The clinical history and the radiological picture generally raise suspicions. Ultrasound examination may detect a variable volume of mediastinal fluid surrounded by inflammatory tissue of moderate to increased echogenicity. The margins are poorly defined and the extent of tissue involvement is often ill defined (Figure 9.6). In some cases the volume of fluid which is noted ultrasonographically does not correlate with what is assumed from the radiographic features. This is more often due to a combination of inflammatory tissue and fluid rather than just fluid alone and is one of the great advantages of ultrasound over radiography.

Pulmonary consolidation

Generally with inflammatory or infectious conditions the lung lobes retain a sharp and almost triangular appearance. This is seen especially clearly where the lung is surrounded by pleural fluid. Unfortunately, consolidated lung has an appearance very similar to that of the liver. Care must be taken to differentiate the two and to correctly interpret mirror-image artefact. In consolidated lung there are small irregular hyperechoic area, which correspond to small pockets of remaining gas (Figure 9.7 a & b). This should

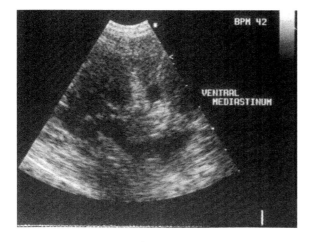

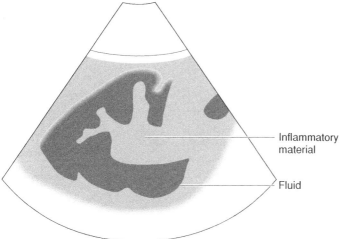

Inflammatory
material

Fluid

Figure 9.6
Mediastinitis in a dog.
Ill defined anechoic
areas sit within areas
of mixed echogenicity
throughout the
mediastinum in this
patient. The whole
area is poorly defined.
This lack of definition
helps differentiate
inflammation from
neoplasia.

help differentiate lung from liver. It is also useful to remember that mirror image artefact does not occur in the face of pleural effusion and that liver tissue should contain characteristic vessels.

Pulmonary consolidation may be due to infection, inflammation, granuloma formation or neoplasia. When assessing an area of consolidated lung tissue, as elsewhere in the body there are certain questions to be asked, which will help produce a list of differential diagnoses: what is the echogenicity; is it homogeneous or is it not and, if not, what echogenicities are present; what shape is the lobe and are the changes discrete?

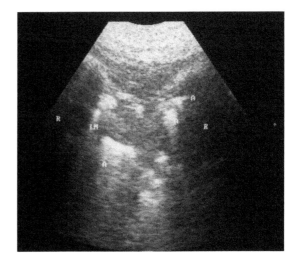

(a)

Figure 9.7 a & b
Consolidated lung *vs.*
mirror-image artefact.
Consolidated lung
tissue can be difficult
to differentiate from
mirror-image artefact.
In consolidated lung
there are often small
pockets of gas
remaining, seen as
small hyperechoic
areas which cast an
acoustic shadow. The
mirror-image artefact
does not show these
features. (R = rib, A =
air, Lm = lung mass.)

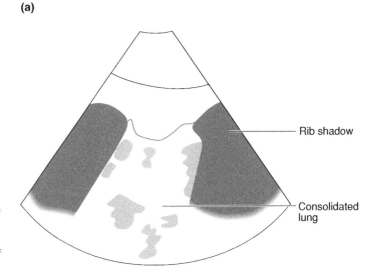

Rib shadow

Consolidated
lung

Pulmonary masses are usually rounded in appearance and
may be hypoechoic, hyperechoic of moderate echogenicity
or mixed. It is not unusual to see an anechoic central region
consistent with necrosis (Figure 9.8). In some cases these
can be difficult to differentiate from abscess formation and
needle-aspirate biopsies must be carefully positioned to avoid
spillage of this material into the thoracic cavity. Additionally,
this material is less likely to contain viable cells and so
is less useful diagnostically anyway. It is not possible to

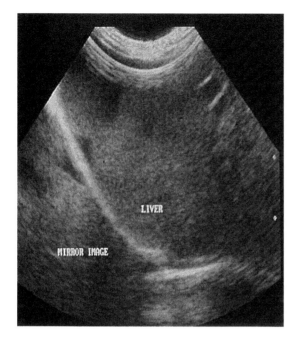

(b)

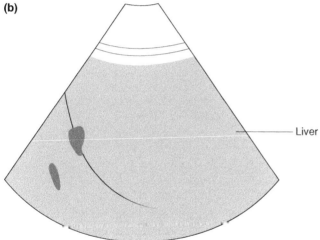

Liver

Figure 9.7 a & b
(*continued*)

differentiate the various pulmonary masses, but in general, tumours are more likely to have a hypoechoic appearance while granulomas are perhaps more likely to be of moderate echogenicity. In some cases tumour infiltrate is more diffuse rather than having a focal or discrete appearance. This

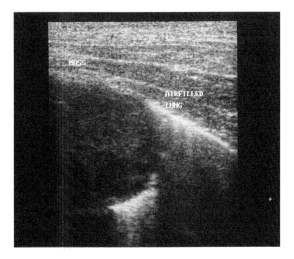

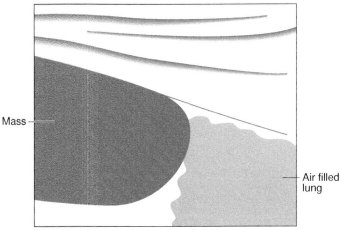

Figure 9.8 The pulmonary tumour seen here is a rounded hypoechoic structure which is well demarcated. The surrounding lung tissue is well defined. This is an appearance commonly seen with pulmonary tumours but may also be seen with granulomas.

Mass

Air filled lung

can be difficult to differentiate from bronchopneumonia except that with inflammation/infection the lung lobe is perhaps more likely to retain a sharp lobed appearance, while some tumour infiltrate produces lung lobes which are rounded and irregular. This detail can only really be appreciated if there is pleural effusion (Figure 9.9 a & b).

Disrupted diaphragm

When looking for diaphragmatic rupture it is important that one can distinguish mirror-image artefact from herniated liver lobe. Remember that mirror-image artefact is not seen

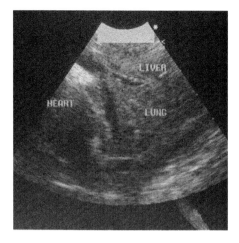

(a)

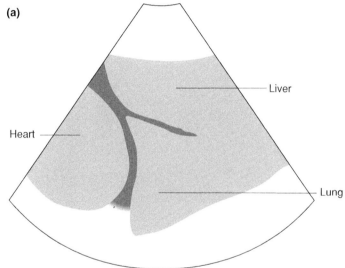

Liver

Heart

Lung

Figure 9.9 a & b
Pulmonary
consolidation *vs.*
pulmonary neoplasia.
(a) Bronchopneumonia
in a cat. This image
shows consolidated
echogenic lung. Note
the small volume of
free fluid. The lung
edge remains smooth
and the tip of the lung
is sharply pointed.

when there is a pleural effusion. It is useful to scan the liver
if entrapment has been longstanding and also to scan the
abdomen to assess what remains in position. This may make
it somewhat easier for the surgeon and is especially relevant
in the case of a long-standing entrapment where, if there is
liver damage, this may affect future prognosis.

The actual defect in the diaphragm may be seen if large
enough, but if small may remain obscured. However,
generally the presence of intestine or other abdominal content on the thoracic side of the diaphragm should indicate

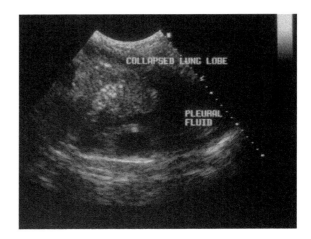

(b)

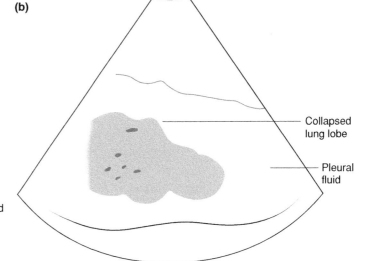

— Collapsed
lung lobe

— Pleural
fluid

Figure 9.9 a & b (b)
Alveolar carcinoma in
a cat. The consolidated
lung is surrounded by
free fluid and has a
rounded and irregular
border.

disruption, although an acoustic window is required to allow
this (Figure 9.10). This may be provided by the herniated
organs or by any free pleural fluid, which may have accumulated as a result. The liver may appear small. If the liver
lobes are entrapped, the tissue is more likely to have an
increased echogenicity and the edges may have become
rounded as a result. The various forms of diaphragmatic
disruption (hernia, rupture or pericardioperitoneal hernia)
cannot be differentiated by ultrasound alone and this is done
on the basis of clinical history and radiographic appearance.

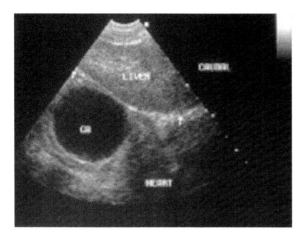

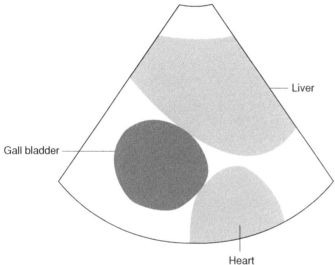

— Liver

Gall bladder ——

Heart

Figure 9.10
Diaphragmatic
disruption. In this
young Cocker Spaniel
with a congenital
diaphragmatic hernia,
the gall bladder (GB)
is seen adjacent to
the heart and on the
thoracic side of the
liver. It is difficult in
many cases to
visualise the defect in
the diaphragm.

Thoracic body wall

Lesions of the thoracic body wall are mainly neoplastic and
the majority arise from the ribs as either chondrosarcoma or
osteosarcoma (Figure 9.11). The benefit of ultrasound is
to allow a clearer definition of the extent of the mass, which
is important for surgical planning and this is especially the
case where there is a considerable volume of free pleural
fluid as a result.

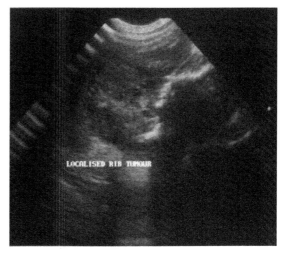

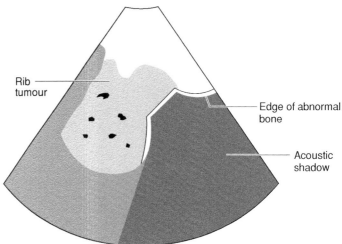

Figure 9.11 Rib tumour. Belgian Shepherd dog with a chondrosarcoma. There is a notable soft tissue component to the tumour and the full extent of the mass can be visualised with ultrasound. The irregular appearance to the diseased rib can also be seen.

Rib tumour

Edge of abnormal bone

Acoustic shadow

Biopsy procedures

In most instances, needle or core biopsy techniques are of benefit in conjunction with transthoracic ultrasound, as they provide a minimally invasive way of providing a presumptive diagnosis and directing the case management. In most cases needle-aspirate biopsies are adequate and certainly would be the technique of choice for a pulmonary lesion. Even with this fairly non-invasive technique there is still a risk of pneumothorax developing as a result of the procedure. It has been suggested that a potentially threatening pneumothorax would develop within the hour and a survey radiograph is recommended one hour following the biopsy to assess for this. While many needle aspirate biopsies may be performed on an outpatient basis, these patients should be hospitalised for the rest of the day or overnight. Core biopsies may be taken of larger mediastinal masses but it is important that these are taken with colour Doppler guidance so that the mediastinal vessels can be avoided.

Suggested reading

Barr, F., Gruffyd-Jones, T., Brown, P. J. & Gibbs, C. (1987) Primary Lung Tumours in the Cat. In: *Journal of Small Animal Practice*, **28**, pp. 1115–1125.

Konde, L. J. & Spaulding, K. (1991) Sonographic Evaluation of the Cranial Mediastinum in Small Animals. In: *Veterinary Radiology and Ultrasound*, **32**, pp. 178–184.

Miles, K. G. (1988) A Review of Primary Lung Tumours in the Dog and Cat. In: *Veterinary Radiology and Ultrasound*, **29**, pp. 122–128.

Stowater, J. L. & Lamb, C. J. (1989) Ultrasonography of Non-Cardiac Thoracic Diseases in Small Animals. In: *Journal of American Animal Hospital Association*, **193**, pp. 514–520.

Teske, E., Stokhof, A. A., van der Ingh, T. S. G. A. M., *et al.* (1991) Transthoracic Needle-Aspiration Biopsy of the Lung in Dogs with Pulmonic Disease. In: *Journal of the American Animal Hospital Association*, **27**, pp. 289–294.

Chapter 10

Imaging the Heart

Johann Lang

Note abbreviations for all figures in this chapter will be found in Table 10.1, p. 215.

Imaging procedure

Thoracic radiography is an excellent method for assessing the size and shape of the cardiac silhouette, as well as for evaluating the pulmonary and great vessels, the opacity and structure of the lung, and the pleural space. Evaluation of the internal architecture and function of the heart using radiography is only possible through invasive contrast procedures.

Echocardiography, on the other hand, provides this information accurately and non-invasively. Two-dimensional (2-D) echocardiography produces real-time, cross-sectional images of the heart and great vessels and allows differentiation of the blood-filled lumen from the soft tissue structures of the heart chambers, valves and vessels. M-mode imaging allows quantitative analysis of the dimensions and motion of chambers and valves; Doppler analysis provides information on the dynamics of the blood flow through the heart chambers, along vessels and across the valves. A thorough cardiovascular examination does not rely solely on echocardiography but includes a detailed physical examination, as well as survey radiography and electrocardiography.

Ultrasound machines and transducers designed for echocardiography allow 2-D (B-mode), M-mode and Doppler examination. Ideally, electrocardiography and Doppler examination, preferably both colour and spectral, are available as concurrent features and most support duplex (or triplex) imaging. This technique makes it possible to display 2-D and Doppler or M-mode images simultaneously using the real-time, 2-D image as a guide for the other modalities. Both modalities are recorded simultaneously. The examination may be recorded on videotape as a sequence of frames with individual frames captured using X-ray film or photographic paper.

Narrow rib spaces and lung surrounding the heart result in relatively small acoustic windows. The ideal transducer therefore should have a small footprint, allowing coupling of the transducer between ribs and producing a wedge-shaped beam which fans out from the thoracic wall. Sector or phased array transducers are therefore the recommended choice for cardiac sonography. The frequency of the transducer depends on the size of the patient and the type of examination. For most dogs both 2-D and M-mode examinations require a 5 MHz transducer. Dogs weighing more than 50 kg may require lower frequencies (3 to 3.5 MHz) whereas small dogs and cats can be examined with a 7.5 MHz transducer. Doppler examinations are usually carried out using lower frequencies than the concurrent 2-D imaging.

In most cases the echocardiographic examination is performed without sedation. In uncooperative patients where sedation is required, it should be remembered that most drugs have potential effects on heart rate, contractility and size. This must be considered during interpretation.

Normally, an area of haircoat is clipped between the costochondral junction and the sternum on both sides of the thorax in the area of the right and left parasternal windows. This may not be necessary in animals with a thin hair coat and the examination may be carried out satisfactorily by preparing the hair coat with surgical spirit and liberal use of coupling gel.

Although the exact placement of the transducer varies between individuals, three main transducer locations or acoustic windows have been described which allow reproducible and consistent image planes. Although the right parasternal window can be found anywhere between the third and sixth intercostal spaces on the right, it is found most frequently in the fourth and fifth spaces, ventrally between the sternum and the costochondral junction. For the left caudal or apical parasternal window, the transducer is placed in the fifth to the seventh intercostal space and as close to the sternum as possible (ideally over the apex of the heart). For the left cranial parasternal window, the transducer is placed in the third or fourth intercostal space between the sternum and the costochondral junction. Otherwise, feel for the apex beat of the heart from the chest wall and use this as a guide for clipping. The subcostal and the suprasternal locations do not allow imaging of the heart in all patients and the following descriptions therefore are limited to the three main windows.

Echocardiography is best performed with the animal placed in left and right lateral recumbent positions on a table allowing transducer placement and examination from the dependent side thus minimising interference from the air-filled lung. Cut-out table tops may be placed on top of the normal table top or a specially designed table produced. However, animals may also be examined in standing, sitting or sternal positions. Patients in heart failure with respiratory distress may not tolerate lateral recumbency and the alternative positions may be used. In all positions the acoustic windows, transducer placement and examination technique remain essentially unchanged.

2-D echocardiography

2-D echocardiography produces real-time, cross-sectional images of the heart and great vessels. These images are relatively easy to interpret because they are similar to anatomical sections through the heart. The images obtained depend on the location of the transducer over the heart and the orientation of the beam plane. Recommendations for standards in transthoracic 2-D echocardiographic examinations in dogs and cats have been published, defining imaging planes and terminology similar to the recommendations made by the American Association of Echocardiography (ASE) for humans. Standardised image orientation is also important. In long-axis views, the index marker of the transducer is directed towards the base of the heart, in short-axis views towards the head of the patient. This image is then displayed with the marker on the right side of the monitor so that the patient's head is displayed on the left and tail on the right.

From each transducer location several different views can be obtained. The name of a specific view or image plane includes the transducer location and the orientation of the image plane relative to the axis of the heart (left ventricle and aorta). A right parasternal long-axis view therefore is obtained from the right parasternal transducer location with the image plane parallel to the left ventricle; for right parasternal short-axis views the plane has to be perpendicular to the long axis of the heart. More detailed specifications include the region of the heart such as papillary muscle or mitral valve or the number of chambers in a specific section such as left caudal parasternal four-chamber view.

M-mode echocardiography

M-mode echocardiography uses a single, thin ultrasound beam rather than a fan-shaped beam, and is used to record and analyse thickness and motion of the soft tissue structures of the heart (heart chamber walls, valves, vessels). The distance of individual structures from the transducer is displayed on the vertical axis and time is displayed on the horizontal axis. M-mode examinations are carried out almost exclusively from the right parasternal approaches. Because most ultrasound machines allow simultaneous recording of B- and M-mode images, placement of the ultrasound beam is made easier by using the real-time 2-D image for orientation. Recognition of specific structures and interpretation is based on a standardised imaging technique, knowledge of the anatomy of the heart and standardised measurements.

Echocardiography is always performed in combination with electrocardiography thus allowing quantitative analysis of measured dimensions, motion and velocities in a standardised way at predefined locations of the time-activity curve of the electrocardiogram (ECG). The measured data may then be correlated with body weight or body surface area and can be compared with normal standards.

The echocardiographic examination must be performed in a standardised way. Images are first taken from the right parasternal location with the animal in right lateral recumbency before proceeding to the left caudal and cranial parasternal locations with the left side dependent.

Normal appearance

Examination from the right parasternal window

Long-axis views

The ultrasound beam is directed parallel to the long axis of the heart and normally two views are obtained. The four-chamber view shows both ventricles, atria and atrioventricular valves and by slight clockwise rotation or angling the ultrasound beam in a cranial direction, the left ventricle outflow tract is displayed with the left ventricle, aortic valve and

Long-Axis 4-Chamber View

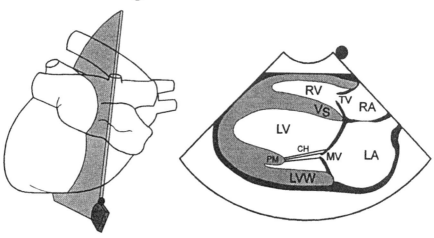

Long-Axis LV Outflow View

Figure 10.1 Diagrams of long-axis views, taken from right parasternal window. Reprinted with permission from Thomas W. P., *et al.* (1993) Recommendations for standards in transthoracic two-dimensional echocardiography in dogs and cats. *J Vet Intern Med*, **7**, 247–252.
For abbreviations see Table 10.1, p. 215.

aortic root. The ventricles are displayed on the left side of the monitor with the atria or aorta on the right side (Figures 10.1, 10.2 a & b).

Short-axis views

From the long-axis view, the transducer is rotated 90° in a clockwise direction and the ultrasound beam is orientated perpendicular to the long axis of the ventricles. Proper

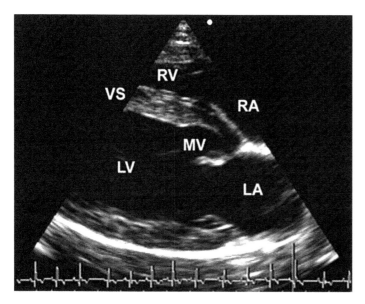

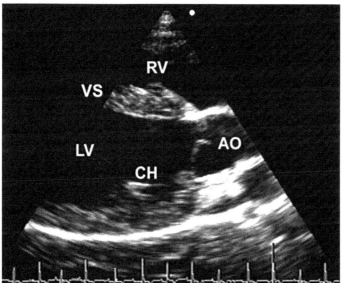

Figure 10.2 a & b
Right parasternal
long-axis views. Figure
(a) corresponds to the
long-axis 4-chamber
view of Figure 10.1.
Diastole: the leaflets of
the mitral valve (MV)
are open. Figure (b)
corresponds to the
long-axis outflow view
of Figure 10.1.
Diastole: the aortic root
(AO) including the
cusps of the closed
aortic valve is
demonstrated. Chordae
tendineae are also
seen.

alignment is achieved if the left ventricle and the aortic root
are displayed as round structures. The examination normally
begins at the level of the apex of the heart, followed by
planes through the papillary muscles, chordae tendineae,
mitral valve, aortic root, left atrium (M-mode) and main
pulmonary artery. For these views, the transducer is angled
progressively from ventral to dorsal, towards the heart base.
The view through the papillary muscles is described as having

Short-Axis Views

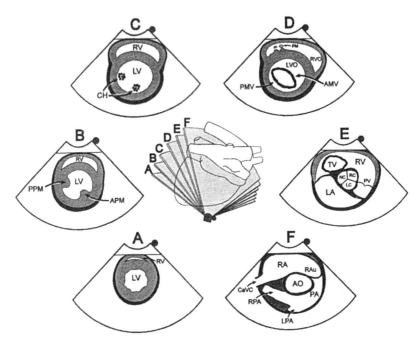

Figure 10.3 Diagrams of short-axis views, taken from right parasternal window. Sections A to F show views at the level of the apex (A), papillary muscle (B), chordae tendineae (C), mitral valve (D), aorta (E), and pulmonary artery (F). Reprinted with permission from Thomas W. P., *et al.* (1993) Recommendations for standards in transthoracic two-dimensional echocardiography in dogs and cats. *J Vet Intern Med*, **7**, 247–252.
For abbreviations see Table 10.1, p. 215.

a mushroom shape, while the view through the mitral valve is known as the fish mouth view (Figures 10.3, 10.4 a, b & c).

Examination from the left caudal parasternal window

Several short- and long-axis, two- and four-chamber views have been described from this transducer location. The most important are the four-chamber, or inflow, view and the five-chamber, or outflow, view. After placement of the transducer over the apex, the ultrasound beam is directed almost perpendicular to the sternum and parallel to the long axis of the heart. By rotating the ultrasound beam in a left caudal to right cranial direction and angling dorsally towards the base of the heart, a four-chamber view is obtained showing the left ventricle and atrium on the right side and the right ventricle and atrium on the left side. The ventricles should

(a)

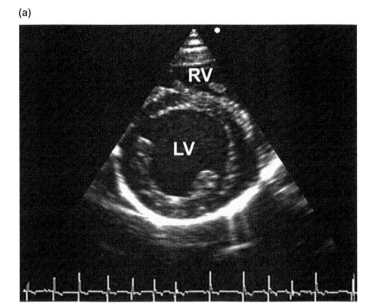

(b)

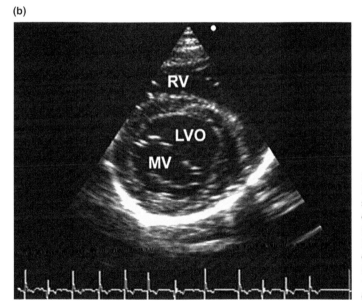

Figure 10.4 a, b & c
Right parasternal
short-axis views. (a)
corresponds to plane B
(papillary muscle) of
Figure 10.3, (b)
corresponds to plane D
(mitral valve) of Figure
10.3. These are
diastolic views.

be displayed 'end on' with the atria in the far field. There is
a great deal of individual variation in the appearance of
these structures, depending on the exact position of the
acoustic window (Figure 10.5, Figure 10.6). By tilting the
ultrasound beam slightly cranially, the left ventricular outflow tract can be displayed between the left ventricle and a
portion of the right atrium (five-chamber view).

(c)

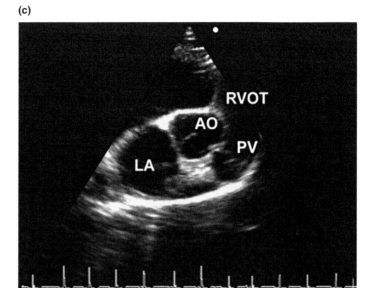

Figure 10.4 a, b & c
(c) corresponds to
plane E (aorta) of
Figure 10.3.
For abbreviation, see
Table 10.1, p. 215.

Figure 10.5 Diagram
of four-chamber or
inflow view, taken from
left caudal parasternal
or apical window.
Reprinted with
permission from
Thomas W. P., *et al.*
(1993) Recommenda-
tions for standards in
transthoracic two-
dimensional echo-
cardiography in dogs
and cats. *J Vet Intern
Med*, **7**, 247–252.
For abbreviations see
Table 10.1, p. 215.

4-Chamber (Inflow) View

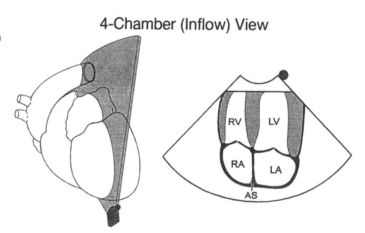

M-mode echocardiography

Echocardiographic measurements are based on 2-D or M-mode images. With good image quality and consistent technique there is a good correlation between the two methods. Cardiac measurements are made routinely and in a standardised way and these recommendations have been published elsewhere. Common measurements made using M-mode include the left atrium/aorta ratio, thickness of the left ventricle free wall and interventricular septum, the internal dimensions of the right and left ventricle in diastole and systole,

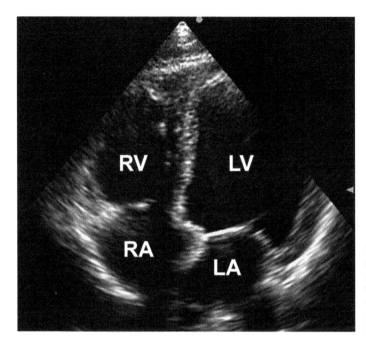

Figure 10.6 Left caudal parasternal or apical window with four-chamber or inflow view in diastole. The plane corresponds to Figure 10.5.

and comparing the aorta and main pulmonary artery (Figure 10.7). Many other measurements are described but are not used routinely and are beyond the scope of this book.

Contrast echocardiography

Contrast echocardiography is a procedure which is only occasionally used to demonstrate malformations of the heart. Due to their special acoustic properties, most currently known echocontrast agents are based on fluid-filled microbubbles. Saline or dextrose mixed with a few drops of the patient's blood, agitated immediately before intravenous injection is a very simple method for studies of the right heart and pulmonary arteries. Because these microbubbles are removed from the blood by the capillary system of the lung, studies of the left heart require more advanced contrast agents. Commercially available liquids or suspensions containing microbubbles based on albumin micro-encapsulated particles or galactose microparticles can survive the pulmonary transit and allow studies of the left heart and the arterial vascular bed.

After an injection of echocontrast into a peripheral vein, the bubbles appear on the 2-D image as small echogenic

Figure 10.7 M-mode recording from a normal dog at two different levels, both taken from the right parasternal location. The vertical axis represents distance from the transducer (top of the image), with the time on the horizontal axis, thus displaying motion of the walls of the heart chambers over time. For the recording to the left, the beam was directed between the papillary muscles at the level of the left ventricular chamber (Figure 10.4 a). During systole the septum and LVW move toward each other. The image to the right was made with the cursor at the level of the mitral valve (Figure 10.4 b). The M-shaped motion of the anterior and the W-shaped motion of the posterior leaflets during diastole are displayed. From M-mode recordings standardised measurements of the walls, heart chambers, aorta and functional parameters are derived.

For abbreviations see Table 10.1, p. 215.

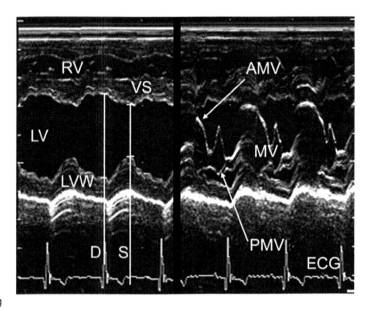

dots, first in the right atrium and then within the right ventricle and main pulmonary artery. The appearance of any echogenic bubbles in the left ventricle, after an injection of echocontrast into a peripheral vein, is a clear sign of a right-to-left shunt. Contrast echocardiography remains the most sensitive method for detecting even small right-to-left shunts. A left-to-right shunt occasionally produces a negative contrast effect adjacent to the defect in the contrast-filled right ventricle. However, non-selective contrast echocardiography is not a reliable method to demonstrate these shunts. These require selective injection of a contrast medium into the left ventricle under general anaesthesia and therefore constitute an invasive method. Contrast studies can be combined with M-mode or Doppler echocardiography thus enhancing the sensitivity of the method.

Echocontrast agents are considered to be very safe as they are well tolerated by patients and no clinically relevant changes in cardiovascular function or permanent complications have been observed. To avoid the risk of air embolism in pulmonary or systemic arteries, care is taken not to inject visible air bubbles.

Doppler echocardiography

It is beyond the scope of this book to cover Doppler echocardiography in detail. It provides extremely valuable and important information on the dynamics of normal and abnormal blood flow through the heart chambers, vessels and across the valves in a non-invasive way.

Several different types of Doppler ultrasound are described. Spectral Doppler is divided into pulsed-wave Doppler and continuous-wave Doppler. On most echocardiographic machines the Doppler frequency shift is displayed as velocity (cm or m/s) but produces also an audible signal. Doppler recordings are displayed with velocity on the y-axis and time on the x-axis, flow towards the transducer above and flow away from the transducer below the baseline. Pulsed-wave Doppler can accurately localise abnormal blood flow and discriminate laminar and turbulent flow where this is of low velocity or is superficial in location, whereas continuous-wave Doppler can measure very high velocities at depth, as seen in cases of pulmonic or aortic stenosis. Pulsed-wave Doppler measures at a specific location using a gate while continuous-wave Doppler measures indiscriminately along its path. Colour-flow Doppler is based on the pulsed-wave Doppler signal and produces a colour-coded image of the mean blood flow velocities. It is laid over the 2-D or M-mode image, mapping the direction, velocity (or velocities) and quality of the blood flow within the area of interest. Using the colour Doppler image as a guide it is very easy to direct the pulsed wave (PW) or continuous wave (CW) to the location with the abnormal blood flow.

Abnormal appearance

Congenital heart disease

Many specific congenital defects are suspected from physical examination of the patient, survey radiographs of the thorax and ECG tracings. However, echocardiography remains the only non-invasive method to diagnose definitively a specific lesion and quantify the severity of the cardiac change. Most congenital heart diseases are based on specific anatomical defects which can be directly demonstrated by sonography. In other cases, the compensatory dilatation or hypertrophy may suggest a specific lesion. Together with the physical examination and radiography, not only the type of defect, but also the severity of the disease can be evaluated – both basic criteria required to establish a prognosis and to give recommendations for a specific therapy (medical or surgical). Because many congenital diseases have a hereditary background, breeding programmes are also often based on the results of an echocardiographic examination. In this chapter only the most common congenital heart defects in dogs and cats are described.

Patent ductus arteriosus (PDA)

Patent ductus arteriosus (PDA) is the result of a failure of the fetal ductus venosus to close after birth and while it is reportedly the most common congenital heart defect in the dog, it is uncommon in the cat. Skilled sonographers are able to visualise a PDA from the left cranial parasternal long-axis view in about 75% of dogs affected. However, it is the recognition of secondary changes and being able to rule out concurrent defects from the 2-D examination which allows confirmation of the diagnosis of PDA in almost 100% of the cases seen. Where the shunt is small, secondary changes include mild dilation of the pulmonary artery and a mild increase in left ventricular end-diastolic dimension. In larger shunts, volume overload in the lung, left cardiac chambers and aorta to the level of the ductus leads to dilation of the main pulmonary artery and left atrium. The left ventricle is also dilated and may show eccentric hypertrophy. The right ventricle remains normal.

M-mode examination allows analysis of most of the secondary changes. Increased left ventricular end-diastolic dimensions with normal septal and left ventricular thickness indicate eccentric hypertrophy. Exaggerated motion of the interventricular septum is indicative of left ventricular overload. Fractional shortening may be normal or increased but if there is myocardial failure, this is decreased. The left atrium and sometimes the aortic root are also enlarged.

A PDA leads to an abnormal flow pattern within the main pulmonary artery. This can be detected and quantified using Doppler sonography. Detection of the characteristic turbulent flow confirms the diagnosis even where the PDA cannot be visualised.

Pulmonic stenosis (PS)

Pulmonic stenosis (PS) is defined as an obstruction in the right ventricular outflow tract, which results in right ventricular pressure overload. This pressure overload and the resultant secondary change (concentric hypertrophy of the right ventricle) are proportional to the degree of obstruction. In most cases, the stenosis is the result of valvular malformation and infundibular hypertrophy can further obstruct the outflow tract. In the English Bulldog and Boxer, pulmonic stenosis can also be caused by an anomalous left coronary artery. Pulmonic stenosis is more common in the dog than in the cat.

2-D ultrasound can demonstrate most of the features of pulmonic stenosis (Figure 10.8). Mild right ventricular hypertrophy may be difficult to detect, whereas in moderate to severe cases, thickening of the septum, right ventricular free wall and papillary muscles are seen. Flattening of the interventricular septum is present in cases with moderate to severe right ventricular pressure overload. Because of interference from the adjacent lung it can be difficult to image the pulmonic valve directly and precise definition of the defect may not be possible. Thickened and immobile cusps are seen with valvular stenosis and a narrow subvalvular or infundibular region with subvalvular stenosis. This, together with post-stenotic dilation of the main pulmonary artery, helps confirm the diagnosis of pulmonic stenosis. Mild dilatation of the right atrium is often associated with right ventricular hypertrophy or mild tricuspid regurgitation. If marked dilatation of the right atrium is present, tricuspid valve insufficiency or a patent foramen ovale should be suspected and evaluated by contrast echocardiography.

M-mode examination is not usually helpful in the diagnosis of pulmonic stenosis. In moderate to severe cases, concentric thickening of the right ventricular free wall and septum can be seen with paradoxical septal motion towards the left ventricle during systole.

Doppler examination can detect mild stenosis where there are no abnormalities in the 2-D or M-mode examination. Pulsed-wave Doppler is used to localise the narrowing and continuous-wave Doppler is then used to quantify the severity by determining the systolic peak velocity and pressure gradient between the right ventricle and pulmonary artery. Prognosis and therapy depend on the severity of the disease and therefore on Doppler measurements. Pressure gradients of less than 50 mm Hg are classified as mild whereas gradients of greater than 125 mm Hg are classified as severe cases. The latter usually require therapeutic intervention. However, the best candidates for balloon valvuloplasty are dogs with gradients of greater than 75 mm Hg.

(a)

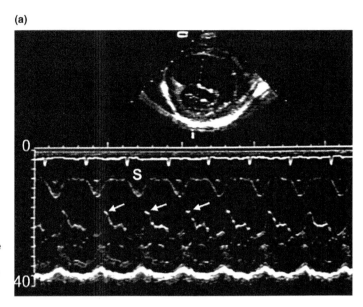

Figure 10.8 a & b
(a) Right parasternal long-axis (four-chamber) view in a dog with congenital pulmonic stenosis. The right ventricle shows concentric hypertrophy with the thickened septum bulging towards the left ventricular chamber.
(b) Same dog as (a) showing continuous-wave Doppler recording from the pulmonary outflow tract and main pulmonary artery. This is a right parasternal short-axis view. There is a systolic high velocity blood flow (5 m/sec ≈ pressure gradient of 100 mmHg) away from the transducer (signal below the baseline) caused by the pulmonic stenosis and a diastolic low velocity signal toward the transducer (above the baseline) caused by pulmonic insufficiency.

(b)

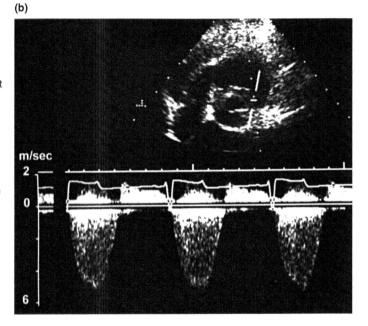

Aortic stenosis (AS)

Aortic stenosis (AS) is defined as an obstruction of the left ventricular outflow tract leading to left ventricular pressure overload. As elsewhere, the pressure overload and concentric hypertrophy are proportional to the degree of obstruction. Complications include left ventricular dysrhythmia and myocardial ischaemia caused by the higher demand and impaired coronary blood supply. In more than 95% of cases, the stenosis is subvalvular in location (SAS). Valvular stenosis is less commonly seen and supravalvular stenosis is extremely rare. Aortic stenosis is the second most common congenital heart defect in the dog and has been reported in the cat.

Mild cases of aortic stenosis may be difficult to detect using 2-D echocardiography. In moderate to severe cases, the left ventricular hypertrophy and the subvalvular stenosis are readily recognised. In the right parasternal short-axis view, narrowing between the interventricular septum and the base of the anterior leaflet of the mitral valve are the main features of subaortic stenosis. Depending on the angle of interrogation and the type of obstruction this appears as a hyperechoic ridge or ring-like structure in the left ventricular outflow tract. In the valvular form, short, thickened and immobile cusps may be present. Post-stenotic dilatation is usually present in animals over six months of age and is best recognised in the right and left long-axis views. Ischaemia with fibrosis may mean that the papillary muscles are hyperechoic when compared with normal musculature. Other features include mild thickening of the mitral valves, mild dilation of the left atrium and abnormal motion of the mitral valves.

M-mode examination shows diastolic thickening of the left ventricular free wall and interventricular septum (concentric hypertrophy) with normal fractional shortening.

Doppler echocardiography can detect mild stenosis with no clear abnormalities in 2-D or M-mode examinations, localise (pulsed-wave Doppler) and quantify the stenosis (continuous-wave Doppler). Prognosis and therapy depend on the severity of the disease and any complications which may be present. Pressure gradients of less than 50 mm Hg are classified as mild, between 50 and 75 mm Hg as moderate and greater than 75 mm Hg as severe.

Ventricular septal defect (VSD)

Most often, ventricular septal defects (VSDs) consist of a single opening in the upper ventricular septum (fibrous) just below the aortic valve on the left (subaortic) and the supraventricular crest (infracristal) beneath the septal tricuspid leaflet on the right side. VSDs in the muscular ventricular septum or more cranial regions of the upper ventricular septum are relatively rare. VSDs are relatively common in dogs and cats and may occur in combination with other defects. A VSD usually results in a left-to-right shunt predominantly during systole with quick ejection of the blood into the pulmonic artery, thus sparing the right ventricle from volume overload. In large defects right ventricular overload and dilatation of the right ventricle, left atrium and left ventricle will occur. Over time, increased pulmonary blood flow may cause increased pulmonary vascular resistance, hypertension and bidirectional or right-to-left blood flow.

With the exception of very small defects, 2-D echocardiography using the right parasternal long- or short-axis plane usually will demonstrate the typical subaortic-infracristal defects. Other locations may require other transducer locations as well. The typical features include left ventricular overload, a hyperdynamic left ventricle and dilatation of the left atrium. In patients with combined VSD and aortic insufficiency, displacement of the right coronary cusp toward the right ventricle may be seen. Contrast echocardiography is very useful to demonstrate right-to-left shunting but of limited sensitivity in left-to-right shunts. Detection of a left-to-right shunt depends on the presence of a negative contrast effect within the right ventricle. B-mode examination is very insensitive in the detection of the defect. It usually demonstrates left ventricle overload with a hyperdynamic left ventricle function and dilatation of the left atrium.

For detection of VSDs with left-to-right shunting, colour Doppler echocardiography is the most sensitive method. An experienced sonographer will detect nearly 100% of VSDs and will also gain information on the magnitude of a shunt. Location and direction of a shunt can be determined best using colour Doppler technique, the high velocity and turbulent systolic jet can be quantified using continuous-wave Doppler.

Atrial septal defect (ASD)

An atrial septal defect (ASD) can occur in different locations. Sinus venosus defects occur near the junction of the cranial vena cava or the pulmonary veins, ostium secundum defects in the mid portion at or near the foramen ovale, and ostium primum defects in the lower portion of the atrial septum. Isolated ASD and patent foramen ovale (PFO) are rare malformations in the dog and cat. PFO is frequently present in dogs with pulmonic stenosis, ostium primum defects are commonly combined with other defects of the endocardial cushions (deformation of atrioventricular valve valves). Small and moderate sized ASDs without other malformations most often have no clinical significance because the shunt volume, usually from left to right, is low. In larger defects, right atrial and ventricular overload may be present.

Moderate sized and large ASDs are readily detected using 2-D echocardiography. The best imaging planes are the right parasternal long- and short-axis views and the left apical four-chamber view. Care must be taken in the area of the ovalis in the caudal part of the septum. This area of the septum is very thin and often produces no echoes, mimicking an ASD. The ASD has to be present in multiple echo planes and is more likely if the edges of the suspected defect are very echogenic and end abruptly. Contrast echocardiography may be helpful especially in cases with right-to-left or bidirectional shunt but can be misleading as well. The secondary dilatation of the right atrium and ventricle are present with larger defects, and the volume overload in the right ventricle may cause flattening of the ventricular septum during diastole. I-mode examination is insensitive in the detection of an ASD and, in larger defects, usually reveals dilatation with eccentric hypertrophy of the right ventricle; paradoxical septal motion may also be present.

In cases with ASD, Doppler examination in the right parasternal long-axis plane usually shows abnormal blood flow across the septum during systole and diastole. During colour-flow examination of the right atrium, flow between ASD, cranial vena cava and tricuspid insufficiency have to be distinguished. In isolated cases flow is usually directed from left to right; in cases with concurrent PS (dogs) or pulmonary hypertension, a right-to-left shunt may be present.

Mitral valve dysplasia (MVD)

Mitral valve dysplasia (MVD) is one of the most commonly seen congenital heart diseases in the cat. Uncommon in dogs, it affects mainly large breed dogs. Shortened, thickened and redundant leaflets, often combined with shortened and thickened chordae tendineae and abnormal papillary muscles will lead to mitral valve regurgitation (common), stenosis (uncommon) or both. MVD is often combined with other abnormalities of the heart, especially in cats. The main

Figure 10.9   Right
parasternal long-axis
view in a dog with
congenital dysplasia of
both atrioventricular
valves. All four heart
chambers are
enlarged. Because
of the dilatation, the
septum and the left
ventricular wall appear
thin. The septal leaflets
of the tricuspid and
mitral valves appear
short. Differential
diagnoses from this
B-mode image include
dilated cardiomyopathy
and endocardiosis with
bilateral atrioventricular
insufficiency.

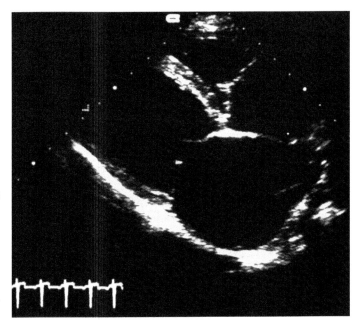

pathophysiological mechanism is volume overload of the left atrium and left ventricle with elevated left atrial pressure. Severely affected animals finally will develop myocardial failure.

The main features of MVD, the often markedly enlarged left atrium and the dilatation of the left ventricle, are easily recognised using 2-D or M-mode echocardiography (right parasternal views) (Figure 10.9). The wall thickness of the left ventricle usually appears normal (eccentric hypertrophy), the contractility depends on the severity and duration of the disease. The shortening fraction may be normal, increased in moderate to severe MVD, or decreased in cases with myocardial failure. Thickened valves with decreased mobility, thickened and short chordae and upwards displaced papillary muscles are best recognised using 2-D echocardiography.

Doppler examination using the left parasternal apical transducer location (four-chamber view) confirms mitral regurgitation or stenosis; colour Doppler is especially helpful in the localisation of small or eccentrically directed, usually turbulent, jets.

Tricuspid dysplasia

Similar to MVD, tricuspid valve dysplasia affects cats and large breed dogs (Labrador Retriever and German

Shepherd dogs) and leads to tricuspid regurgitation. The pathophysiology is similar to MVD. Dilatation of the right atrium with diastolic flattening of the ventricular septum are the main features, best seen using 2-D echocardiography.

Tetralogy of fallot

Tetralogy of Fallot (TOF), although rare in dogs and cats, is the most commonly encountered complex malformation in the dog and cat and consists of following abnormalities:

1 ventricular septal defect
2 pulmonic stenosis
3 right ventricular hypertrophy and
4 dextraposition (overriding) of the aorta. VSD and PS are pathophysiologically important, leading to right ventricular hypertrophy and in cases with severe pulmonic stenosis to a right-to-left shunt.

The typical features of 2-D echocardiography from the right parasternal locations include concentric hypertrophy of the right ventricle, the usually large VSD and the overriding aorta. It is important to evaluate the pulmonic valve (TOF typically has valvular stenosis) and main PA allowing differentiation of TOF with persistent truncus arteriosus (no separate PA) and Eisenmenger's syndrome (right-to-left shunt without pulmonic stenosis). M-mode echocardiography is especially helpful in assessing the concentric hypertrophy, but fails to demonstrate all the features of a TOF.

Non-selective contrast echocardiography, by injecting echocontrast into a peripheral vein allows documentation of right-to-left shunting. The echogenic bubbles are first observed in the right ventricle and can be traced across the VSD into the left ventricle.

Eisenmenger's syndrome and other malformations

Eisenmenger's syndrome, a communication between the right and the left side of the heart (at the level of the atria, ventricular septum (VS) or great vessels), pulmonary hypertension and right-to-left shunt and many other malformations are described in the dog and cat. It would be beyond the scope of this book to describe these rare congenital deformities. Most of them can be diagnosed correctly by a skilled cardiologist or radiologist using echocardiography, but some may also require cardiac catheterisation and contrast studies.

Acquired heart disease

The echocardiographic examination of acquired heart disease follows the same principles as for congenital heart defects. The first step is to recognise secondary abnormalities such as dilatation or hypertrophy of heart chambers. Second, identification of the primary lesion is important and third, comparison of the echocardiographic findings with the clinical examination, ECG and radiographs. In this section, degenerative and infective valvular disease, myocardial and pericardial diseases are described.

Degenerative valvular disease

Endocardiosis (myxomatous degeneration), a degenerative disease of the endocardium may lead to mitral and/or tricuspid insufficiency, but rarely to stenosis. Involvement of the mitral valve and tricuspid valve is very common, the aortic valve rarely, and the pulmonic valve is almost never affected. Uncommon in cats, it affects mainly older small to medium-sized dogs. Irregular thickening, especially at the ends of the leaflets which are unable to close at systole, sometimes combined with elongated or ruptured chordae tendineae cause insufficiency of the affected valves. Similar to MVD, the main pathophysiological mechanism of acquired mitral valve insufficiency is volume overload of the left atrium and left ventricle.

The echocardiographic findings associated with endocardiosis are similar to MVD (see p. 205): abnormally thickened, isoechoic or hypoechoic leaflets and often markedly enlarged left atrium and the dilatation of the left ventricle at diastole (eccentric hypertrophy) are easily recognised using 2-D echocardiography (Figure 10.10). M-mode echocardiography (right parasternal short-axis view) often underestimates dilatation of the left atrium, but readily identifies the other features including exaggerated septal motion. Increased shortening fraction, due to compensatory systolic myocardial function, is typically observed until late in the course of the disease and the finding of a normal or decreased shortening fraction should be considered a sign of myocardial failure. Prolapse of the leaflets into the atrium is a sign of ruptured chordae tendineae and often leads to a sudden worsening of the regurgitation.

Doppler examination using the left parasternal apical transducer location (four-chamber view) confirms mitral or

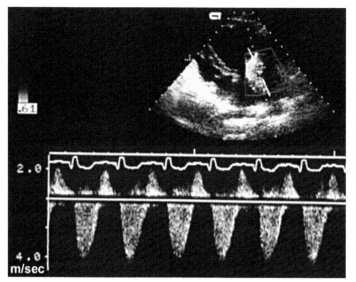

Figure 10.10 Chronic degenerative mitral valve disease (endocardiosis) in a dog. Continuous-wave Doppler recording of the left inflow tract in a left apical four-chamber view, demonstrates high velocity flow from the left ventricle back into the left atrium (away from the transducer: below the baseline).

tricuspid regurgitation. Colour Doppler is especially helpful in the localisation of small or eccentrically directed, usually turbulent, jets and for placement of the sample volume for spectral analysis.

Similar to degenerative mitral insufficiency, tricuspid insufficiency mainly affects dogs and leads to tricuspid regurgitation. Dilatation of the right atrium and right ventricle and increased motion of the right ventricle during systole, as well as flattening of the septum during diastole (paradoxical septal motion) in severe cases are the main features of tricuspid insufficiency, best seen using 2-D echocardiography.

Infective endocarditis (IE)

Bacterial infection caused by septic thrombi affect mainly the mitral valve and/or aortic valve, rarely the tricuspid valve and pulmonic valve. Although the most common cause of acquired aortic insufficiency, the condition is rare in dogs and cats. Infective endocarditis causes insufficiency of the affected valves, left ventricular overload and left heart failure (Figure 10.11).

In cases with IE, 2-D echocardiography readily identifies the shaggy appearance or the hyperechoic irregular vegetations at the normally thin aortic cusps. Mitral valve vegetations may be more difficult to be distinguished from chronic endocardiosis even more so because the secondary changes of the heart are also similar to other causes of mitral regurgitation.

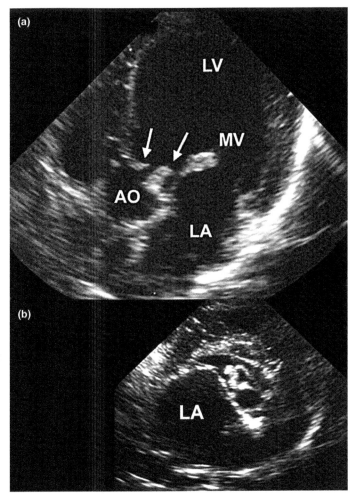

Figure 10.11
(a) Left apical view in a dog with infective endocarditis. Very irregular and hyperechoic nodular vegetations are present on the aortic and mitral valves. These have resulted in aortic and mitral insufficiency. In the short-axis view (b) the thickened cusps of the aortic valve appear as very hyperechoic and irregular structures in the outflow tract.

Colour Doppler (left or right long-axis views) and spectral Doppler echocardiography (left apical long axis) can be made and easily confirm regurgitation of the aortic valve and mitral valve. The typical feature of aortic valve insufficiency is the turbulent jet from the aortic valve into the right ventricle during diastole. Systolic velocities in the aorta are usually normal.

Cardiomyopathy

Myocardial dysfunction can be caused by many different factors. Disorders secondary to valvular insufficiency or stenosis, shunts or other diseases have been discussed earlier.

This paragraph discusses primary disorders described as dilated or hypertrophic cardiomyopathy. Dilated cardiomyopathy (DCM) mainly affects large to giant breed dogs and became a relatively rare condition in cats after supplementation of the amino acid taurine in canned cat food. Hypertrophic cardiomyopathy (HCM) affects cats but seems to be extremely uncommon in dogs. In the cat restrictive and unclassified forms of myocardial diseases are also described. In addition to these primary myocardial disorders, X-linked muscular dystrophy in the dog and cat and hyperthyroidism are also known causes of myocardial dysfunction.

Dilated cardiomyopathy describes a condition which includes hypokinesis with reduced ejection and shortening fractions, diastolic and systolic dilatation of the affected ventricle, dilated atria and finally congestive heart failure. In cats and dogs it may affect both ventricles, or only the left ventricle in some dogs. M-mode and 2-D examinations readily identify these features even in milder forms of DCM and are very helpful in the differentiation of primary myocardial dysfunction from other heart diseases. The dilated chambers, hypokinesis of the mitral valve and left ventricle are easily appreciated using 2-D echocardiography, the increased internal end-diastolic and end-systolic dimensions of the affected ventricle, the reduced shortening fraction, the reduced thickening of the left ventricle and septum during systole can be quantified using M-mode measurements. The echocardiographic features of DCM in cats is similar to the biventricular condition in dog.

Doppler echocardiography is helpful to identify and estimate the severity of the mitral valve or TCV insufficiency, which causes additional volume overload of the left atrium.

Hypertrophic cardiomyopathy usually describes primary concentric hypertrophy of the left ventricle, which leads to decreased left ventricular compliance and impaired diastolic function. It may or may not be associated with mitral valve insufficiency but is often associated with thrombo-embolism of the left side of the heart and arteries.

Typical features of HCM in cats are thickening of the septum and left ventricular wall, which may be symmetric or asymmetric, and left atrium (Figure 10.12). Other features include asymmetric septal hypertrophy, left ventricle dynamic outflow obstruction and abnormal anterior motion of the sometimes thickened mitral valve leaflets during systole. The right side of the heart also may be affected. M-mode and

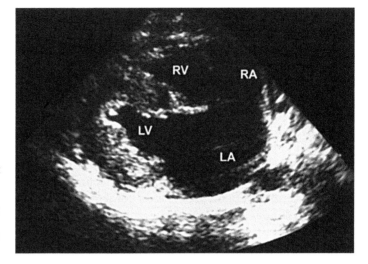

Figure 10.12 Right parasternal long-axis view of a cat with hypertrophic cardiomyopathy in diastole. Both the right and left ventricles are compromised by the concentric hypertrophy of the ventricles, and both atria are severely enlarged.

2-D echocardiography usually readily identify these features – although it is important to image the heart in several planes using 2-D echocardiography because of the great variability of the hypertrophy. In the left atrium or left ventricle, thrombi may be seen. M-mode measurements quantify the reduced left ventricle internal diameter, Doppler echocardiography may be helpful to detect and quantify dynamic outflow obstruction and MV regurgitation. The main features of restrictive cardiomyopathy are diastolic dysfunction of the left ventricle without detectable hypertrophy and uni- or bilateral atrial dilatation.

Hyperthyroidism in cats may cause changes similar to those described for HCM but with increased diastolic dimension of the left ventricle, increased shortening fraction and dilatation of the aortic root.

Pericardial disease

Pericardial effusion (PE) is the most common pericardial disease in dogs and cats and may or may not be associated with cardiac tamponade. Cardiac tamponade occurs when the pericardial pressure is higher than the intracardiac diastolic pressure leading to decreased filling of the ventricle, decreased stroke volume and impairment of the venous return. Because of the relatively thin wall of the right ventricle, clinical signs of right heart failure are usually present. In cats, where pericardial diseases with tamponade are less common than in dogs, feline infectious peritonitis and tumours

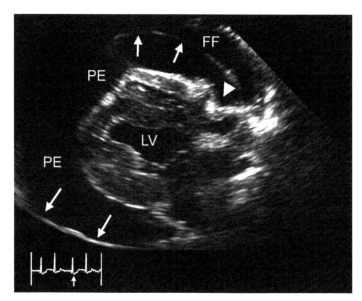

Figure 10.13 Right parasternal long-axis view of a dog with idiopathic pericardial effusion (PE) and cardiac tamponade. The white arrows point to the distended pericardial sac. In diastole, a large effusion is compressing the right atrium (arrowhead). The left ventricular chamber appears small. Free fluid (FF) in the pleural space is also present.

(lymphosarcoma) are the most common causes. In dogs, PE with cardiac tamponade are often caused by tumours of the right atrium (haemangiosarcoma), heart base and pericardium, idiopathic pericarditis and left atrium rupture.

In cases with cardiomegaly, echocardiography is the method of choice in differentiating primary heart disease from pericardial effusion and in searching for the cause of the effusion. The 2-D examination is very sensitive detecting even very small amounts of fluid in subclinical cases. Due to the effect of gravitational forces, scans from 'below' the animals are more sensitive. Features of pericardial effusion include a hypo- or anechoic space between the heart wall and pericardial sac. In more pronounced cases, diminished right ventricle and left ventricle internal dimensions and swinging of the heart in the fluid-filled pericardial sac (bizarre motion in the M-mode examination) during the heart cycle are present. Diastolic collapse of the right atrium and right ventricle, best seen in the right parasternal long-axis view, and decreased filling of the left ventricle characterise heart tamponade (Figure 10.13). In cases with pleural effusion, the pericardium can be outlined. In pericarditis or cases with diffuse neoplasia (mesothelioma), the pericardium may be thickened; in cases with haemorrhagic effusion (idiopathic PE, tumour), intrapericardic hyperechoic thrombi may be identified and mistaken for neoplastic masses.

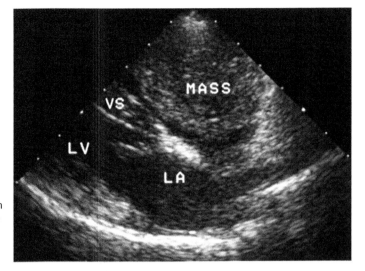

Figure 10.14 Right parasternal long-axis plane in a dog with a large mass arising from the right atrium. In this case the mass was not associated with pericardial effusion but it caused compression of the right atrium with clinical signs of right heart failure.

Right atrium masses, most often haemangiosarcomas, are best imaged from the right parasternal views, but the left cranial views are also important. They arise from the right auricle, right atrium wall or the junction of right atrium and right ventricle, most of them projecting into the pericardial sac. Small cavities often give them an irregular appearance (Figure 10.14).

Heart base tumours (aortic body, ectopic thyroid tumours) originate around the ascending aorta and may grow invasively in any direction and may penetrate the heart wall or chambers. They require multiple-plane imaging from both sides of the thorax and are more homogenous compared to right atrium tumours.

Other pericardial mass lesions include tumours (mesothelioma, lymphosarcoma, others), abscesses, cysts and granulomas. Using 2-D echocardiography they may readily be detected if concomitant PE is present. In most cases mesotheliomas lead to diffuse thickening of the pericardium and/or epicardium without clear masses and cannot be distinguished from inflammatory disorders sonographically.

Constrictive pericarditis is a rare condition leading to thickened and fibrotic pericardium with reduced ventricular filling. In cases without PE the abnormal pericardium may be difficult to detect. A thickened and hyperechoic pericardium may be present in 2-D echocardiography and a flattened left ventricle diastolic wall motion on the M-mode image.

Other acquired heart diseases

Cor pulmonale, caused by acute or chronic pulmonary hypertension (dirofilariosis, other causes of pulmonary artery (PA) occlusion, severe parenchymal lung disease or hypoxia), leading to RV enlargement, produces usually eccentric hypertrophy of the RV and considerable dilatation of the main PA and its branches. These changes, including secondary tricuspid and PA regurgitation, are readily detected using 2-D and Doppler echocardiography.

Table 10.1 Abbreviations for all figures in Chapter 10.

AMV	Anterior mitral valve cusp		•	Transducer index mark
AO	Aorta		PM	Papillary muscle
CaVC	Caudal vena cava		PMV	Posterior mitral valve cusp
CH	Chorda tendinea		PV	Pulmonic valve
D	Diastole		RA	Right atrium
ECG	Electrocardiogram		RAu	Right auricle
LA	Left atrium		RC	Right coronary cusp
LC	Left coronary cusp		RPA	Right pulmonary artery
LPA	Left pulmonary artery		RV	Right ventricle
LV	Left ventricle		RVOT	Right ventricular outflow tract
LVO	Left ventricular outflow tract		S	Systole
LVW	Left ventricular wall		TV	Tricuspid valve
MV	Mitral valve		VS	Ventricular septum
NC	Non-coronary cusp			

Suggested reading

Boon, J. (1998) *Manual of Veterinary Echocardiography*, 1st edn, Lippincott Williams & Wilkins, Hagerstown, MD.

Fox, P. R., Sisson, D. & Moise, N. (1999) *Textbook of Canine and Feline Cardiology: Principles and Clinical Practice*, 2nd edn, pp. 159–160. W.B. Saunders Co., Philadelphia.

Nyland, T. G. & Mattoon, J. S. (2002) *Small Animal Diagnostic Ultrasound*, 2nd edn, Chapter 18: 'Echocardiography.' pp. 354–423. W. B. Saunders Co., Philadelphia.

Thomas, W. P., Gaber, C. E., Jacob, G. J., *et al.* (1993) Recommendations for Standards in Transthoracic Two-dimensional Echocardiography in Dogs and Cats. In: *Journal Veterinary Internal Medicine*, 7, pp. 247–252.

Chapter 11

Doppler Ultrasound

Johann Lang

Before the imaging procedure can be described, it is imperative that the principles and physics behind Doppler ultrasound are fully understood. These are described below.

Indications

Doppler Ultrasound is an important part of every echocardiographic examination in animals being screened for or with suspected cardiac disease. While B-Mode technique is used for examination of the normal and abnormal anatomy of the structures of the heart, Doppler ultrasound is used for describing and measuring normal and abnormal blood flow (direction, velocity and spectral pattern) within the heart and through atrioventricular, pulmonic and aortic valves.

Doppler ultrasound examinations include investigation of blood flow in arteries and veins in almost each body part. Examples are suspected thrombo-embolic disease processes in the aorta, caudal vena cava, mesenteric vessels and parenchymatous organs such as spleen, liver or the kidneys. Calculation of flow indices (e.g. resistive index in kidney disease) are based on Doppler measurements and give important diagnostic and prognostic information. Investigation of normal and abnormal splanchnic blood flow, suspected portosystemic shunt, arteriovenous abnormalities, investigation of tumour vascularisation or tumour infiltration into vessels (e.g. in adrenal tumours) are other indications. It would be beyond the scope of this book to list all indications described. More details are listed in the respective chapters of the different organ systems.

Principles

In 1842, Christian Doppler published the theory that the frequency of a wave changes between a moving wave source and the target. Based on the shift of the sound frequency of

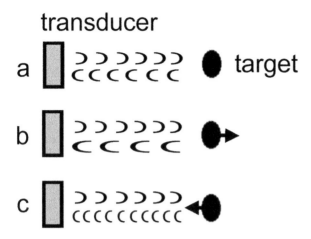

Figure 11.1 Doppler effect. If the source of sound waves (transducer) and the target are stationary, the frequencies to and from the target are the same (a). A target moving away from the source (b) causes a downward shift, a target moving towards the source (c) causes an upward shift in the frequency of the returning sound waves.

a moving train, a stationary listener can decide whether a train is approaching or receding. With an approaching train the sound becomes louder as it approaches (positive Doppler shift) and reduces as it moves away (negative Doppler shift). Were the listener to move at the same speed as the train, the sound would not change as there is no longer a Doppler shift. The Doppler effect also occurs if radio waves are reflected from a moving target like a flying aircraft. In other words, the effect of shifting sound frequency occurs whenever the distance between the sound source and the receiver changes with time. In a contracting space, the sound waves are compressed; in a distracting space, they are stretched (Figure 11.1). In medical ultrasound, the ultrasonic Doppler effect occurs usually between a stationary transducer transmitting and receiving sound and the blood cells as moving reflectors. In this situation, the waves travel from the source to the receiver by reflection. Movement of the reflector towards the transducer causes a positive or upward shift of the received ultrasound wave frequencies and movement away produces a negative or downward shift of the received ultrasound wave frequencies. The Doppler shift frequency can be calculated as follows (Figure 11.2):

$$f_D = 2 \cdot f v_r \cos\Theta / c$$

where f_D is the Doppler shift frequency, f the transmitted frequency and v_r the velocity of the moving erythrocytes. Θ represents the angle of interrogation and if this is 90° the cosine of this is 0. This poses a problem because many of the vessels to be imaged lie at 90° to the ultrasound beam

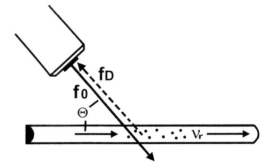

Figure 11.2
Illustration of the
Doppler formula:
$f_D = 2f_0 v_r \cos\Theta/c$.

and as such poor results are achieved. This can be circumvented by scanning from different angles and with the patient in different positions. For greatest accuracy the angle of interrogation should be less than 60°. The factor 2 occurs in the equation because the sound waves are compressed twice, first by the receiving erythrocytes moving toward the transducer and again between the reflecting erythrocytes and the transducer. In medical applications there is almost always an angle between the transducer and the blood vessel. Therefore, according to the rules of trigonometry, we have to correct our result with $\cos\Theta$; c is the velocity of speed in tissue. The Doppler shift frequency usually lies within the audible range and can be displayed using loudspeakers or the video monitor, where the Doppler shift frequency or the (computed) velocity is displayed on the vertical axis and time on the horizontal axis.

For medical imaging, mainly two types of Doppler ultrasound are used: pulsed-wave and continuous-wave Doppler. Colour-flow Doppler ultrasound is also used extensively for echocardiography and abdominal imaging. Power Doppler is a more recent development and is used mainly in abdominal or small-part imaging where low blood velocities are encountered. Power Doppler is not available on all machines. A full description of this is beyond the scope of this book.

Pulsed-wave Doppler

The principle of pulsed-wave Doppler is similar to B-mode imaging where sound is transmitted in short pulses and received by the same crystal during the time interval between emission of pulses. By setting the sample volume in a vessel at a specific depth, the echoes returning from this vessel will arrive after a specific time interval. This time interval corresponds to the depth of the vessel (called range gating) and allows blood flow in a specific vessel to be measured. In this way, the location of a flow pattern can be precisely determined. The size of the gate is usually called the sample volume and can be adapted for the size of the vessel. In this technique only one crystal is used for transmitting and receiving sound and the depth of pulsed-wave Doppler, as well as the measurable velocities, are limited. In order to measure blood-flow velocity correctly, the pulse repetition frequency must be twice the highest frequency of the returned echoes (known as Nyquist limit). When the Nyquist limit is exceeded an artefact known as aliasing occurs which makes accurate interpretation of the flow velocity impossible. This will occur where the pulse repetition frequency is too low or where there is high velocity flow such as in aortic or pulmonic stenosis or where the depth of sampling is too great. In these cases it will be necessary to change to continuous-wave Doppler ultrasound instead.

Continuous-wave Doppler

In this technique sound is transmitted and received continuously. The transducer contains two crystals, one which transmits and the other which receives sound. Sound waves are therefore received continuously and so continuous-wave Doppler (CW Doppler) can measure very high velocities but is unable to discriminate the depth of the signal. Every moving target in the path of the sound beam will cause a signal and will be measured. The origin of the measured velocities must be localised using pulsed-wave Doppler (spectral or colour-coded). CW Doppler is used to measure flow velocities in animals with heart disease associated with high speeds of flow such as aortic or pulmonic stenosis, ventricular septal defects or mitral and tricuspid insufficiency (Figures 10.8b, p. 202, 10.10, p. 209).

Duplex Doppler, colour Doppler, power Doppler

Ultrasound machines with phased array and linear array transducers allow the cursor and sample volume to be placed using the B-mode image as a guide and also to record a B-mode image simultaneously with the Doppler spectrum (duplex Doppler). In contrast, when using a mechanical transducer, the B-mode image will be frozen. In colour Doppler, the Doppler mean shift frequencies in a specific area are measured, colour coded and superimposed over the 2-D greyscale image. Direction and velocities of flow in a large area can be displayed using different colours for the direction and velocity of flow, e.g. red, orange, yellow for flow towards the transducer, blue and green for flow away from the transducer. The lighter hues usually indicate greater speeds. Mapping a wide area makes interpretation and identification of normal and abnormal flow easier but on the other hand, colour Doppler only measures mean velocities and the maximum velocity is limited.

Imaging procedure

The imaging procedure will vary between individuals in an attempt to gain most accurate displays, but there are standard approaches to the major vessels interrogated. If colour Doppler is available, the vessel in question can first be localised and identified using colour Doppler and the direction and character of the blood flow analysed. Precise measurement of blood-flow velocity and characterisation (analysis of Doppler spectrum) of blood flow is done by switching to pulsed-wave and/or continuous-wave Doppler. Two methods are described to measure blood-flow velocities within a vessel: the uniform insonation method where the sample volume is larger than the diameter of the vessel and the maximal velocity method with a small sample volume placed in the centre of a vessel. Using the latter method, the measured velocity has to be multiplied by a factor of 0.57 to determine the mean blood-flow velocity. Position and angle of the transducer has to be adjusted in order to keep the Doppler angle below 60°. Larger angles will not give reliable measurements. It is also important to control the pressure applied with the transducer upon the vessel, because flow will change considerably if vessels are compressed during investigation. Doppler examinations are recorded on videotape for analysis. Interrogation of individual vessels is described in the respective chapters.

Interpretation

The understanding of different waveforms is crucial if using Doppler ultrasound as a diagnostic tool. The spectrum of

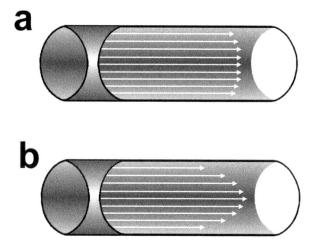

Figure 11.3 Blood-flow velocity profiles vary with vessel size: (a) in larger arteries (e.g. aorta, Figure 11.4) a plug profile indicates that nearly all erythrocytes travel at a similar speed. (b) Smaller vessels (e.g. renal artery, Figure 11.5) have a more parabolic flow profile indicating that the speed of the erythrocytes gradually decreases from the centre to the periphery of the vessel.

the Doppler shift frequencies, usually plotted with velocity on the vertical axis of the display (time on the horizontal axis), depends on the flow profile and whether it is laminar or turbulent, but also on the method used. In larger arteries with undisturbed blood flow, a plug-flow profile is typical whereas parabolic-flow profiles are typical of smaller vessels (Figures 11.3, 11.4, 11.5, 11.8, p. 224). These profiles are explained by the fact that blood in the centre of a vessel flows faster than near the wall. The spectrum of returned frequencies therefore will be broader in a small artery or vein compared to the spectrum of the aorta. The displayed spectrum also depends on whether a small sample volume is placed in the centre of a vessel measuring only the fastest velocities in the centre, or a large sample volume encompassing the entire vessel measuring also the slow velocities near the vessel wall. Disturbed, turbulent flow will be shown as very broad spectrum compared to a narrow spectrum reflecting laminar flow.

The flow patterns in echocardiography have been described and three typical of these are shown here (Figures 11.6 a & b, 11.7). The flow profiles of the aortic and pulmonic outflow tracts and inflow into the right ventricle are similar to the profiles shown herein. The flow profiles in major vessels of the abdomen have also been described. Normal profiles of the abdominal aorta, the renal and coeliac artery pre- and post-prandial (Figures 11.4, 11.5, 11.8), the caudal vena cava, the portal and hepatic vein are shown (Figures 11.9, 11.10, 11.11). The mesenteric artery has a similar profile to

Figure 11.4 Normal pulsed-wave Doppler spectrum of the abdominal aorta in a dog. The recording is taken near the renal artery (r) with a small sample volume ('I' within aorta) in the centre of the vessel measuring only the fastest velocities. Flow towards the transducer is displayed above the baseline as velocity (m/sec). The waveform is typically triphasic with peak systole (P); early diastolic flow reversal (E) and the decreasing diastolic forward flow (D). The narrow envelope enclosing a well defined spectral window (W) is a sign of laminar blood flow with a 'plug profile' indicating that all erythrocytes are travelling nearly at the same speed.

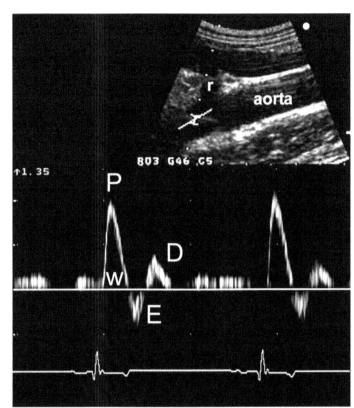

Figure 11.5 Normal pulse-wave Doppler spectrum of the left renal artery in a dog. Spectral broadening without a spectral window indicates a parabolic flow profile, typically for smaller arteries, where the erythrocytes at the periphery of the vessel travel at a slower speed compared to the erythrocytes in the centre of the vessel. A low resistance pattern with a gradually decreasing high diastolic forward flow (D) is typical of an artery supplying the parenchyma. The systolic peak (P) is broad with early systolic peak.

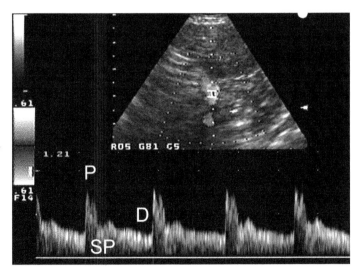

(a)

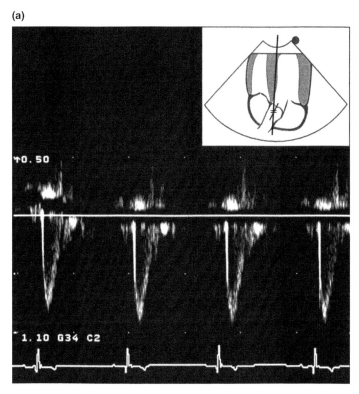

(b)

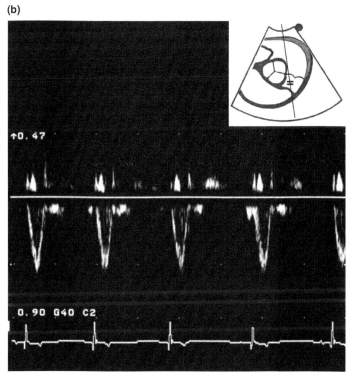

Figure 11.6 a & b
Normal pulsed-wave
Doppler spectrum of
the aortic root (a),
taken from the left
apical parasternal
window and pulmonic
trunk (b), taken from
the right parasternal
window (transducer
location). In both
vessels the sample
volume is placed distal
to the semilunar valves
(see line drawing).
Flow away from the
transducer is displayed
below the baseline (B)
as velocity (m/sec).
The pulsed-wave
spectra of both vessels
are similar with a
narrow envelope
enclosing a well
defined spectral
window (W) as a sign
of laminar blood flow
with a 'plug profile'.
The very high
acceleration of blood
flow within the aorta is
displayed as the
almost straight left part
of the Doppler curve
compared to the
almost symmetric
systolic curve in the
pulmonic trunk.
Immediately distal to
the semilunar valve
there is normally no
diastolic flow present.

Figure 11.7 Normal pulsed-wave Doppler spectrum of the inflow from the left atrium into the left ventricle in a dog. The sample volume is placed within the ventricle just below the mitral valve. Flow towards the transducer is displayed above the baseline as velocity in m/sec. The waveform typically is biphasic with an E- and A-wave. The E-wave is higher compared to the A-wave and reflects passive inflow of blood into the left ventricle after the opening of the atrioventricular valves. At the beginning very fast, the flow slows down as the pressure in the atrium rises. The A-wave reflects active inflow because of atrial contraction.

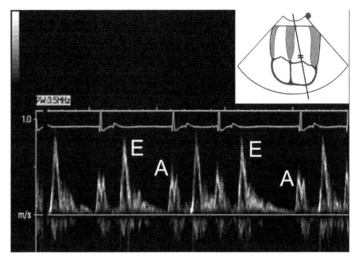

(a)

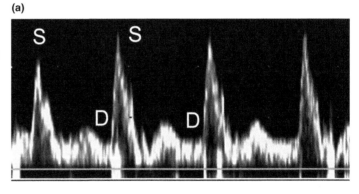

(b)

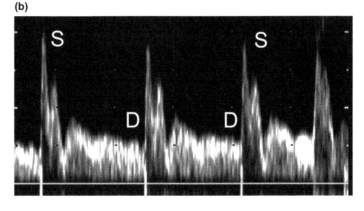

Figure 11.8 Normal pulsed-wave Doppler spectrum of the coeliac artery in a dog in fasted stage (a) and 20 minutes after food intake (b). Before food intake the cranial mesenteric artery shows a high resistance flow pattern with low end-diastolic velocity changing into a low resistance flow pattern 20 minutes after food intake (b) with a higher end-diastolic velocity. The waveform of the post-prandial tracing is similar to vessels serving parenchyma such as the renal artery. The waveform of the coeliac artery and the cranial mesenteric artery are similar (not shown).

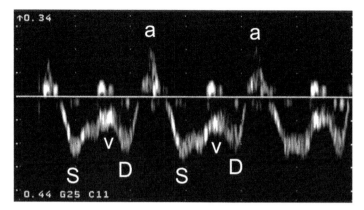

Figure 11.9 Normal pulsed-wave Doppler spectrum of the abdominal caudal vena cava in a dog. The recording is at the level of the liver taken with a small sample volume in the centre of the vessel. Flow away from the transducer is displayed below the baseline as velocity in m/sec. The waveform represents a pulsatile flow with the first antegrade wave (D-wave) during movement of the annulus toward the cardiac apex. It slows down as the pressure in the atrium rises (V-wave). Flow increases again after opening of the tricuspid valves and blood flow from the atrium into the ventricle (D-wave). Flow is reversed during atrial systole (A-wave). An additional retrograde C-wave may be seen when the tricuspid valve closes. Changing intrathoracic and intra-abdominal pressure caused by the respiratory cycle also cause alteration in blood flow velocity.

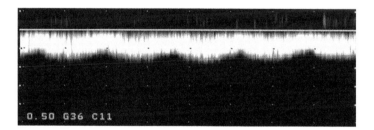

Figure 11.10 Normal pulsed-wave Doppler spectrum of the portal vein at the level of the antrum of the stomach. The wave below the baseline indicates flow away from the transducer. The continuous flow shows only mild undulations representing respiration with higher flow velocities during expiration.

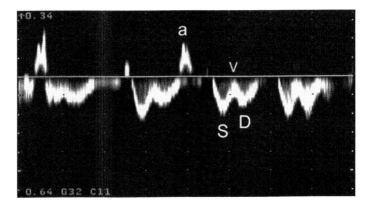

Figure 11.11 Normal pulsed-wave Doppler spectrum of a hepatic vein. Flow away from the transducer in the direction of caudal vena cava is displayed below the baseline (m/sec). The waveform represents a pulsatile flow with augmented flow during atrial diastole (legend analogue to caudal vena cava). After opening of the atrioventricular valve flow increases again. Flow is reversed or stopped during atrial systole.

the coeliac artery with an even lower end-diastolic flow in the fasting stage. After feeding it also changes into a more low-resistance-type flow pattern.

Note that many examinations are not ideal and excessive patient motion, if the patient is uncooperative, or excessive panting, will produce artefact, which makes interpretation more difficult.

Suggested reading

Nyland, T. G. & Mattoon, J. S. (2002) *Small Animal Diagnostic Ultrasound*, 2nd edn, Chapter 2: 'Physical Principles, Instrumentation, and Safety of Diagnostic Ultrasound,' pp. 19–29. W. B. Saunders Co., Philadelphia.

Curry, T. S. III, Dowdey, J. E. & Murry, R. C. (1990) 'Ultrasound,' In: *Christensen's Physics of Diagnostic Radiology*, 4th edn, pp. 323–371. Lea & Febiger, Philadelphia.

Chapter 12

Imaging of the Neck

Alison Dickie

Imaging procedure

Most of the structures within the neck are relatively super-ficial in position, being less than 6 cm below the skin surface. Since the beam is not required to penetrate far, this region should ideally be examined using a high frequency trans-ducer such as 7.5–15 MHz, which will result in high resolu-tion images. This is beneficial since many of the structures in this region are relatively small in size and consequently sonographic changes within them may be more difficult to appreciate using a lower frequency transducer.

A linear transducer is best suited to examination of this region as it provides images with excellent near-field definition, allowing even very superficial structures to be adequately imaged. However, these transducers have a relat-ively large area of contact with the skin surface, which can make them difficult to use in restricted areas such as at the angle of the mandible. For the rest of the neck region this is not a problem and so these remain the transducers of choice. Linear transducers designed for bovine and equine repro-ductive examinations may also be used for examination of this region.

Sector and microconvex or curvilinear transducers have a smaller area of contact with the skin surface but the near field of the image is distorted to varying degrees preventing very superficial structures being adequately imaged. How-ever, this can be alleviated by placing an echolucent stand-off pad between the transducer and the skin surface, moving the area of interest down into the focal zone of the beam and therefore improving the quality of the image obtained. In a practice situation, the choice of transducer will be largely dictated by availability of equipment.

The animal is placed in a position which allows adequate access to the region being examined. This includes lateral, dorsal or sternal recumbency and also standing or sitting positions, although the latter two may result in some degree of patient movement. Dorsal recumbency is probably the most desirable, especially when the entire cervical region is to be examined, as it allows access to all aspects of the neck. This can be achieved by placing the patient on a padded mat or in a radiographic cradle. When firm but gentle restraint is applied, sedation is not usually required unless the patient is particularly fractious or resents being in that position. Cats will more commonly require sedation, particularly if they are hyperthyroid.

If the entire cervical region is to be examined then the skin surface is prepared by clipping the hair from the angle of the mandible to the thoracic inlet on the ventral and lateral aspects of the neck. However, it is often sufficient to clip a smaller region directly over the area of interest if the lesion is more localised. Surgical spirit and then liberal quantities of ultrasound coupling gel are applied to ensure good acoustic contact, thereby improving the quality of the images obtained. If a stand-off pad is used then gel should be placed between the pad and the skin surface and also between the pad and the transducer face to ensure adequate transmission of the beam into the patient.

Familiarity with the anatomy of the region under examination should be obtained by consulting anatomy texts prior to commencing with the examination. The region of interest should be imaged in both the transverse and longitudinal planes from a variety of angles and a series of sweeps made with the ultrasound beam to ensure that the entire structure is imaged. When structures are paired, the contralateral side of the body should also be imaged allowing comparison between normal and abnormal structures, which in many cases will increase the confidence with which abnormalities can be identified. If a lesion is identified, ultrasound can be used to guide interventional techniques such as fine-needle aspirates or biopsies. This is particularly advantageous given the large number of blood vessels within the neck and the close proximity of most structures to them.

Larynx, trachea and oesophagus

Imaging procedure

To image the larynx, a small region of hair is clipped from the ventral aspect of the neck immediately caudal to the angle of the jaw. The thyroid cartilages can be palpated in the midline as the two laminae meet while the cricoid is palpable caudal to this. These are used as landmarks to guide placement of the transducer on to the ventral midline of the neck in a transverse orientation. Sector or linear transducers may be used and imaging is performed in the transverse plane so that both sides of the larynx are visible in each slice allowing comparison and an assessment of the symmetry between the two halves. Rocking the transducer in a cranio-caudal direction allows the entire larynx to be visualised although it may also be necessary to alter to the location of the transducer in a cranial or caudal direction. Care should be taken not to apply too much pressure with the transducer as this can be uncomfortable for the patient. Patience is often required since the procedure commonly stimulates swallowing and subsequent movement of the larynx which may necessitate repositioning of the transducer.

Imaging of the larynx is best performed with the dog in dorsal recumbency as it is easier to maintain the position of the transducer in the middle of the neck, although a sitting position may be better tolerated by the patient. If the transducer slips off to one side of midline then the symmetrical appearance of this structure is lost, which may make it more difficult to identify abnormalities. However, once a lesion has been identified, examination from a series of more lateral locations may be beneficial in further evaluating that region.

The trachea is imaged by maintaining the transducer in the ventral midline of the neck and moving it caudally off the larynx. A more extensive region of hair must be clipped depending on how much of the trachea is to be imaged and it can be followed caudally from the larynx to the thoracic inlet maintaining its mid-line location. It can also be imaged in the longitudinal plane by rotating the transducer through 90° in addition to a series of more lateral locations to ensure the entire structure has been evaluated fully.

The oesophagus originates dorsal to the trachea and then runs along the left side of the trachea to the level of the thoracic inlet. It maintains a position dorsolateral to the trachea for most of the length of the neck.

Normal appearance

The ultrasound beam will not penetrate gas so the air within the lumen of the larynx produces a hyperechoic region on the image with a marked distal acoustic shadow. This is usually associated with reverberation artefacts which produces a 'sunbeam' type of appearance. The contour of this hyperechoic line will vary depending on the shape of the soft tissue–air interface which the beam encounters, but nothing beyond it can be imaged making it impossible to visualise the dorsal aspect of the larynx.

In a cranial location, the base of the epiglottis can be imaged as a curved hyperechoic line. Caudal to this, the ventral aspect of the thyroid cartilage, which is located between the transducer and the air-filled lumen, can be imaged as an inverted 'V' shape extending into the far field. However, the wall itself is poorly visualised due to the detrimental effects on the image of artefacts arising as a result of the close proximity of the intraluminal air. The vocal folds are visualised as hypoechoic, triangular-shaped structures arising from the internal aspects of the lateral walls of the larynx. They are visible because of their soft-tissue nature, which displaces the air from the lumen of the larynx and allows penetration of the beam. The narrow air column between the vocal folds appears as a small hyperechoic region and a thin, vertical reverberation artefact. In real-time imaging, slight abduction or adduction of the vocal folds is evident in a panting animal but little movement may be visible when the animal is at rest. However, the gas column should remain symmetrical and is seen to vibrate during normal respiration. There are two short, hyperechoic lines visible one on each side of midline which represent the arytenoid cartilages (Figure 12.1). Their movement throughout the respiratory cycle is easier to observe than that of the vocal folds and should demonstrate symmetrical abduction during inspiration. Further caudal angulation of the transducer will allow the ventral aspect of the cricoid cartilage to be imaged, which has a more rounded shape. The musculature adjacent to the larynx appears well defined and hypoechoic.

The dorsal aspects of the lateral cartilage, in addition to the dorsal aspect of the larynx, are obscured by the acoustic shadowing produced by the gas and so are not visible. Both sides of the larynx should be symmetrical and the gas should fill the entire lumen except at the level of the vocal folds. Imaging from a more lateral location on the neck allows the side of the larynx nearest the transducer to be better evaluated. However, the far wall is then obscured by the shadowing from the gas and is not visible.

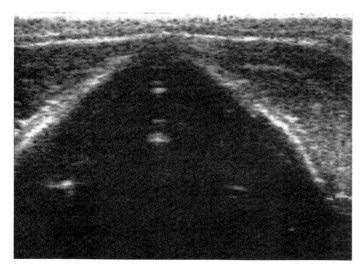

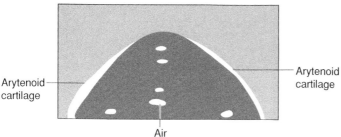

Arytenoid cartilage

Arytenoid cartilage

Air

Figure 12.1 Normal canine larynx. The region of the larynx between the transducer and the air column is visible. The arytenoid cartilages are visible as two short, hyperechoic lines one on each side of midline.

The gas-filled lumen of the trachea produces a curved hyperechoic soft tissue–gas interface due to its rounded shape and again, the distal acoustic shadowing and reverberation artefacts prevent visualisation of the far wall. The lumen is larger in diameter than the larynx but the wall of the trachea itself may be poorly visualised. This is again due to the close proximity of the intraluminal air, producing artefacts which have a detrimental effect on the resulting image quality. When imaged in long axis, the hyperechoic interface is linear and produces a striated appearance which results from the alternate acoustic shadowing from the tracheal cartilage rings and reverberation from the air (Figure 12.2).

The oesophagus is a poorly defined structure and so may be easily overlooked, especially in the cranial cervical region, where it is in a dorsolateral location relative to the trachea and so may be obscured by the intraluminal gas. Further, caudally it may be imaged to the left of the trachea in short axis as an oval or irregular-shaped structure adjacent

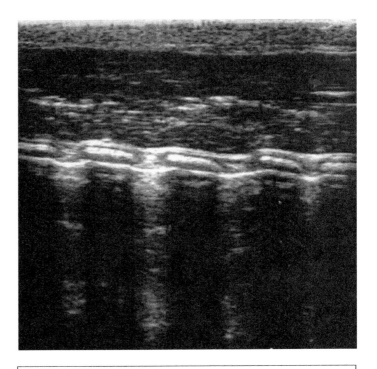

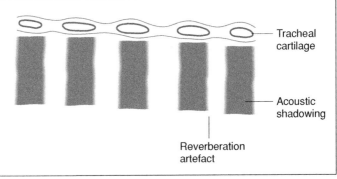

Figure 12.2 Normal trachea. Long-axis image demonstrating hyperechoic sections of the tracheal cartilages and the striated appearance which results from the alternate acoustic shadowing from these and reverberation from the intraluminal air.

Tracheal cartilage

Acoustic shadowing

Reverberation artefact

to the common carotid artery. The walls are hypoechoic while mucus within the lumen may produce a hyperechoic central region possibly producing some shadowing if intraluminal gas is present. In long axis it appears as an indistinct tubular structure containing poorly defined hyperechoic linear streaks resulting from the intralumenal material and so may be difficult to image.

The sonographic anatomy of larynx, trachea and oesophagus in the cat is similar to that of the dog and therefore these structures are imaged in the same way.

Abnormal appearance

Ultrasound can be used to investigate cases of laryngeal paralysis in the dog. There is failure in abduction of the vocal fold on the affected side during inspiration, which produces asymmetry of the air column on the ultrasound image. However, since the normal movement of the vocal folds is relatively small, this may be difficult to assess so it is often useful to also observe the motion of the cuneiform processes of the arytenoid cartilage which appear as distinctive hyperechoic linear structures on either side of midline. The affected side will demonstrate an absence of the normal abduction of this structure on inspiration, resulting in it remaining motionless or moving up and down rather than in a lateral direction.

Ultrasound is also useful to identify masses associated with the larynx in both dogs and cats. If these arise from the internal surface and project into the lumen then they will displace the gas resulting in asymmetry of the air column and will be visualised as echogenic structures. The size of the mass and its location can be assessed but its echogenicity can be very variable and mixed depending on the composition of the mass. If structures such as the vocal cords are displaced then this will result in distortion of the normal laryngeal anatomy. In the presence of marked disruption there is often an absence of normal anatomical features which produces a very confusing appearance. In these cases, movement or vibration of the air column in association with respiration will indicate the location of the lumen. It may not be possible to visualise lesions arising from the dorsal aspect of the larynx due to the intervening air.

Masses projecting beyond the external walls of the larynx will distort the smooth, well defined margins of this structure and any extension to involve adjacent structures can be identified. Masses arising externally may displace the larynx or involve the walls and it may be useful to image from a more lateral location or in a longitudinal plane to determine the extent of the mass. The surrounding area can also be examined for evidence of lymph node enlargement.

Thyroid and parathyroid glands

Imaging procedure

The thyroid gland is a bilobed structure with one lobe on each side of midline. It is located on the ventrolateral aspect of the trachea, caudal to the larynx and extending for approximately the first five to eight tracheal rings. Occasionally the two lobes communicate via the isthmus which spans the ventral aspect of the trachea. The thyroid is surrounded by a thin fibrous capsule.

The thyroid is best imaged with the patient in dorsal recumbency and the neck extended to allow adequate access to the cranial cervical region. The close proximity of the gland to the transducer, especially in cats and small dogs, may necessitate the use of a stand-off, depending on the type of transducer being used for the examination. The transducer is placed in the jugular groove and each lobe of the thyroid is examined in turn by locating the common carotid artery in long axis immediately caudal to the larynx. The transducer is then rocked in a ventromedial direction which allows the thyroid gland to be identified medial to the common carotid artery in its location between it and the trachea. Each lobe is imaged as a thin, well defined, fusiform structure which is hypoechoic relative to the surrounding tissue but more echogenic than the adjacent musculature (Figure 12.3). It is homogenous but surrounded by a thin,

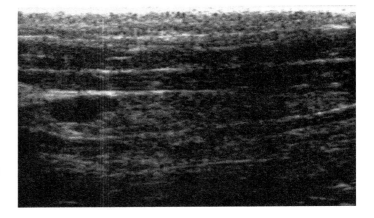

Figure 12.3 Normal canine thyroid and parathyroid glands imaged using 13 MHz transducer. Long-axis view demonstrating thin, fusiform thyroid gland surrounded by a well defined, hyperechoic, fibrous capsule. The cranial parathyroid gland appears to be embedded within the thyroid tissue and is hypoechoic relative to it.

hyperechoic, fibrous capsule. Normal limits for long- and short-axis dimensions of the thyroid have been reported as approximately $5 \times 1.5 \times 0.5$ cm in dogs and 2.0–3 cm long and 0.2–0.3 cm wide in cats. However, the small size of the normal thyroid gland may make it difficult to visualise in all planes unless a high frequency transducer such as 10 MHz is used and so it may not be possible to determine these parameters in all cases.

Both lobes of the thyroid should be examined in a series of imaging planes. In the transverse plane they appear as hypoechoic triangular-shaped structures immediately medial to the common carotid arteries. Occasionally, the cranial and caudal thyroid arteries may be imaged if a high frequency transducer is used. They appear as small, anechoic, tubular structures running from the common carotid arteries towards the thyroid but may be difficult to identify in the absence of Doppler ultrasound to confirm the presence of blood flow within them.

The parathyroid glands in the dog and cat can vary in number and location although there are usually four which are relatively consistent. Two are associated with each thyroid lobe, one caudal which is embedded within the thyroid tissue, and one cranial which is outside the thyroid capsule, although it is embedded within the fascia and so closely associated with it. They are therefore imaged by the same procedure used to image the thyroid gland. The normal parathyroid glands are between 2 and 4 mm in diameter and are less echogenic than the surrounding thyroid tissue. However, unless a dedicated high frequency transducer, such as 10 MHz, is used, normal parathyroid glands are not routinely visualised in the dog and cat (Figure 12.3).

Abnormalities of the thyroid gland

Feline hyperthyroidism

Ultrasound can be useful to investigate the thyroid glands in hyperthyroid cats especially if nuclear scintigraphy is not available. The advantages of ultrasound over other techniques are its widespread availability, low cost, rapidity of performance and lack of harmful effects.

The most common cause of hyperthyroidism in cats is thyroid adenoma or adenomatous hyperplasia. The majority of hyperthyroid cats have glands which are uniformly enlarged and they are therefore much more readily identified than normal glands. They lose their thin fusiform shape, becoming plump or sausage-shaped, and may have undulating margins producing a lobulated appearance. In short axis they lose their triangular shape and become more rounded in appearance. Most tend to remain homogeneous although some may appear mildly mottled and the overall echogenicity can be variable with a tendency to be less than that observed in normal glands. Occasionally, cystic structures may also be identified within these thyroid glands which appear as discrete anechoic regions of varying size with distal acoustic enhancement. They can be located anywhere within the gland and may be single or, more commonly, multiple (Figure 12.4).

Occasionally, unilateral lesions occur in cats resulting in one enlarged thyroid lobe being identified but an inability to image the other. This is due to the resulting atrophy making the gland very small and similar in appearance to the surrounding structures so it therefore becomes extremely difficult to identify. Likewise, ultrasound may not be sensitive enough to identify the presence of ectopic thyroid tissue in other locations within the cervical region due to the disseminated nature of the tissue and the similarity in its appearance to the surrounding soft tissues. This will depend to some extent on the frequency of the transducer.

Thyroid carcinomas

Thyroid carcinomas in the dog and cat commonly cause massive enlargement of the thyroid gland and result in marked distortion of the topography of the region. Therefore, care must be taken to rule out other regional structures as the possible origin of the mass. Failure to identify the normal thyroid gland and the presence of a large mass in its place suggests that the mass is thyroid in origin.

The sonographic appearance of thyroid carcinomas is very variable. Some may be well marginated with a well defined smooth capsule, although most tend to be have poorly defined margins and may extend to involve adjacent tissue (Figure 12.5). They usually have an echogenicity which is less than normal thyroid tissue although they are heterogenous in appearance with a mottled appearance and often contain hyperechoic foci representing fibrous tissue or

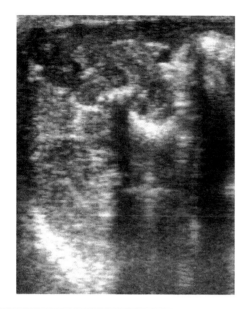

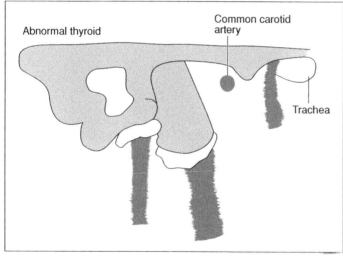

Abnormal thyroid

Common carotid artery

Trachea

Figure 12.4 Thyroid adenoma in a cat. Short-axis view demonstrating a markedly enlarged thyroid gland which has lost its normal triangular shape and is lobulated in outline. In addition there are several small anechoic cystic regions within it and an area of mineralisation. It can be seen surrounding the common carotid artery and extending across midline between the transducer and the trachea suggesting bilateral involvement.

microcalcification. Regional lymph node enlargement may be identified, suggesting that localised metastasis has occurred or the lesion may be visualised invading localised structures such as the oesophagus, common carotid artery or jugular vein. Thyroid carcinomas are usually highly vascular lesions so ultrasound is useful to guide needle placement for aspiration while avoiding the larger vessels.

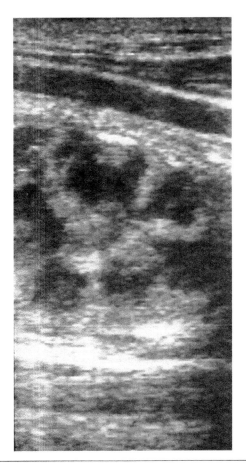

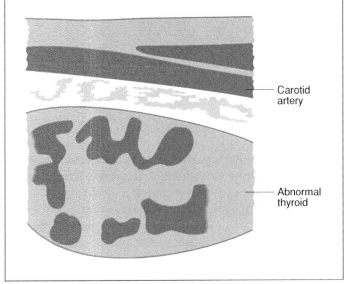

Carotid
artery

Abnormal
thyroid

Figure 12.5 Thyroid carcinoma in a dog. Long-axis view demonstrating well encapsulated mass of mixed echogenicity deep to the common carotid artery with central cystic areas.

Abnormalities of the parathyroid gland

Ultrasonographic examination of the parathyroid glands is a useful procedure in the investigation of hypercalcaemia in cats and dogs. The parathyroid glands can only be imaged using ultrasound if they are sufficiently enlarged or altered in echogenicity for them to become distinct structures and be differentiated from the adjacent thyroid tissue. Primary parathyroid hyperplasia, hyperplasia secondary to chronic renal failure, parathyroid adenomas and carcinomas will usually all result in changes within one of the parathyroid glands rendering it visible on ultrasound. However, hypercalcaemia of malignancy is not associated with any abnormalities within the parathyroids and therefore, in these cases, they will usually remain undetectable on ultrasound examination.

Usually only one parathyroid gland is affected, and the anatomical location of the lesion associated with either the cranial or caudal pole of the thyroid gland usually allows differentiation from thyroid lesions, although occasionally they may be identified within the centre of the thyroid gland. Changes within the parathyroid gland usually result in the development of a round-to-oval-shaped nodule of varying diameter which may be well or poorly defined and, if large enough, may distort the outline of the thyroid gland. These nodules are commonly either anechoic or hypoechoic in echogenicity producing varying degrees of distal acoustic enhancement.

Parathyroid carcinomas are less commonly encountered than adenomas or hyperplasia and may be less well defined in appearance in addition to invading the surrounding tissue. However, it is not possible to differentiate between malignant and benign conditions on the basis of their sonographic appearance alone since, as with most other organs, there is a large overlap in ultrasound findings between different conditions. However, the changes in the parathyroid glands associated with primary hyperplasia or secondary to chronic renal failure rarely cause enlargement of the gland to beyond 5 mm in diameter while the presence of an adenoma or carcinoma will commonly do so. It is therefore sometimes possible to differentiate between these conditions on the basis of size with a nodule of greater than 5 mm diameter suggesting the presence of an adenoma or carcinoma.

It is likely that these parameters also apply to the cat although this has still to be confirmed.

Blood vessels

Imaging procedure

The main blood vessels within the cervical region are the common carotid arteries and the external jugular veins, which are paired vessels each running the length of the neck to either side of midline. The hair from the jugular grooves is clipped to allow imaging of these structures. Each external jugular vein is a superficial structure located just below the skin surface in the jugular groove on the ventrolateral aspect of the neck. The common carotid arteries are deeper structures located lateral to the lobes of the thyroid gland in a lateral and slightly dorsal location relative to the trachea. In the presence of unilateral abnormalities, it may be useful to compare the abnormal with the normal side.

The external jugular vein is imaged by placing the transducer in the jugular groove and should be imaged in both long and short axis. The superficial nature of the jugular vein can make it difficult to image since any pressure on the skin surface with the transducer can result in collapse of the vessel and therefore failure to visualise it. This may be overcome by occluding the vein in the caudal cervical region with digital pressure which will prevent it from collapsing as a result of external pressure, therefore improving imaging of this vessel. An improvement in image quality may also be achieved by using a stand-off pad to increase the distance between the transducer and the vein which will move the structure down into the focal zone of the beam. This is especially the case when using a sector transducer due to the presence of near-field distortion.

The common carotid artery is also imaged by placing the transducer in the jugular groove but this time the beam is angled in a more dorso-medial direction. Its deeper location means that a stand-off pad is not usually required.

Normal appearance

When imaged with the transducer parallel to the long axis of the neck, the external jugular vein appears as a tubular structure with thin hyperechoic walls and an anechoic lumen and can be followed along the full length of the neck. Gentle pressure with the transducer will cause visible compression of the lumen. Rotation of the transducer through 90° to image in short axis results in the vessel becoming oval in shape although the outline will vary depending on the degree of pressure exerted with the transducer. Venous flow within the vessel can be confirmed if Doppler ultrasound is available.

The common carotid artery is also visible as a tubular structure when imaged in long axis with an anechoic lumen and hyperechoic walls. It is of a smaller diameter than the jugular vein but is not compressible and occasionally in real-time imaging, pulsation may be visible. It appears round rather than oval-shaped when imaged in short axis as its thick arterial walls maintain the lumen diameter even in the presence of external compression. The common carotid artery can be followed from the thoracic inlet to the cranial cervical region where it divides to form the smaller internal and larger external carotid arteries. The external carotid artery continues in a similar plane to the common, but the internal leaves in a medial direction before resuming a cranial path. A localised bulge in the walls of the internal carotid artery is visualised where it arises from the common carotid which represents the carotid bulb and can be used to confirm the identity of the vessel.

Appearance of abnormalities

The most important application of ultrasound, when assessing vascular structures in the cat and dog, is to assess their relationship to other cervical lesions. Masses within the neck may distort the normal anatomy and displace the blood vessels, resulting in the vessel being imaged following an abnormal or tortuous route through the cervical region (Figure 12.6). Alternatively, the mass may surround the vessel which is imaged passing through it, although in many cases this causes compression of the vessel resulting in compromise of the lumen diameter. This may make it difficult to differentiate from the surrounding tissue. Loss of the well defined hyperechoic vessel wall within the mass may suggest that invasion of the vessel wall has occurred especially if echogenic material is visualised projecting into the lumen, which may further compromise the lumen diameter or induce thrombus formation. In some cases, Doppler ultrasound may

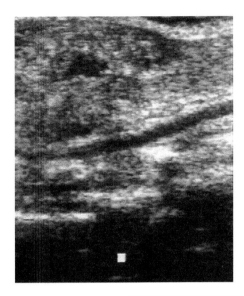

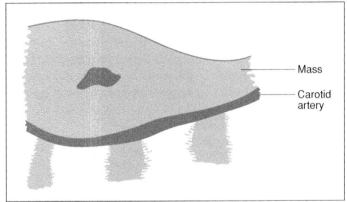

Figure 12.6 Cervical mass in a dog. Long-axis view demonstrating the mass displacing the common carotid artery and compressing the lumen suggesting that the vessel is compromised.

Mass

Carotid artery

be required to identify this compromise by demonstrating variances in the blood flow through the vessel.

It is also usually possible to differentiate between blood vessels and cystic lesions using ultrasound by altering the angle of the transducer. Normal blood vessels will alternate between a tubular branching appearance which can be followed through the cervical region or mass and a round appearance as the beam is rotated from long to short axis, whereas cavitated regions will remain a similar shape when imaged from a variety of angles. However, vessels associated with tumours may be grossly abnormal and so it may not always be possible to differentiate blood vessels and cystic lesions without the use of Doppler ultrasound to detect the presence of blood flow. Identification of major blood vessels within or adjacent to a lesion will help to plan an approach for ultrasound-guided aspirate or biopsy techniques or a surgical procedure.

Jugular catheterisation over a long period may result in thrombus formation arising at the site of the catheter. This will be visible as an elongated hypoechoic structure within the lumen of the jugular vein and Doppler ultrasound will demonstrate either a complete absence of blood flow or marginisation of flow around the structure. In chronic cases, the development of multiple collateral vessels will appear as a series of anechoic tubular structures in the surrounding area. The development of arteriovenous fistulas in the neck is uncommon but will also appear as a series of tortuous, anechoic tubular structures associated with localised bruit.

Lymph nodes and salivary glands

Imaging procedure

The mandibular salivary glands are prominent paired structures which are located in the cranial cervical region under the caudoventral angles of the mandible. Encapsulated within the cranial portion of them is the monostomatic portion of the sublingual salivary gland. The parotid salivary gland is located further cranio-dorsally at the base of the ear. Examination requires clipping in the region of the angle of the jaw and best imaging is achieved with the dog in lateral or dorsal recumbency.

Clipping in this region also allows the retropharyngeal lymph nodes to be imaged in their location close to the mandibular salivary glands, lateral to the common carotid artery and dorsolateral to the larynx. The mandibular and parotid lymph nodes are smaller structures and are therefore not consistently imaged. In addition, there is a series of lymph nodes located throughout the cervical region known as the deep cervical lymph nodes. They are located at a level lateral to the trachea but can be very variable in location and number and so therefore require a larger area of clipping in order to allow examination of the entire cervical region.

Normal appearance

The salivary glands are distinctive structures of low to medium echogenicity with well defined, smooth, hyperechoic

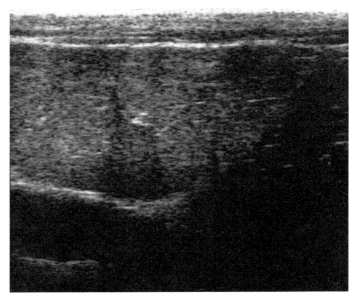

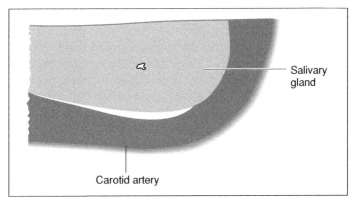

Figure 12.7 Normal mandibular salivary gland. Long-axis image demonstrating its superficial location between the skin and the common carotid artery. It has a well defined, smooth, hyperechoic margin and is of medium echogenicity containing a series of hyperechoic linear streaks representing the fibrous duct system within it.

margins. They contain a series of hyperechoic linear streaks or flecks which represent the fibrous duct system within them (Figure 12.7). The mandibular gland is easy to image in a location superficial to the carotid artery and is oval-shaped but ultrasound cannot readily distinguish it from the adjacent monostomatic portion of the sublingual salivary gland. The parotid salivary gland is less well imaged in its location at the base of the ear.

Normal lymph nodes are identified as oval-shaped or fusiform, hypoechoic structures with well defined smooth margins. The retropharyngeal lymph nodes are relatively consistently imaged and may be 2–4 cm long (Figure 12.8). However, the parotid and submandibular lymph nodes are

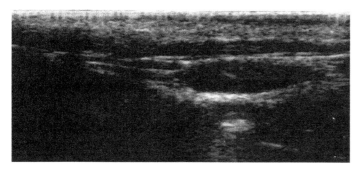

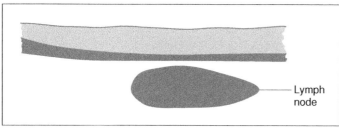

Lymph
node

Figure 12.8 Normal
retropharyngeal lymph
node. Long-axis view
of this fusiform shaped,
hypoechoic structure
with well defined
smooth margins.

not routinely identified as they are usually less than 5 mm
in length and may appear similar in echogenicity to the
surrounding tissue. This is also the case with the deep
cervical lymph nodes which are small in size and have a
variable location resulting in a lack of specific anatomical
landmarks by which to localise them.

Appearance of abnormalities

Enlargement of the lymph nodes makes them much easier
to identify using ultrasound and it is also possible in some
cases to identify non-palpable nodes. The increase in size
observed will vary depending on the underlying process, but
most demonstrate an increase in all dimensions producing a
plump or sausage-shaped structure although the margins
usually remain well defined. They may appear hypoechoic or
hyperechoic as a result of inflammation or infiltration and
may take on a grainy or mottled, heterogeneous appearance.
Although ultrasound provides an accurate method to identify
lymph node enlargement, measure their size and assess their
echogenicity, there is a large degree of overlap between the
appearance and size of reactive, infected and neoplastic lymph
nodes, so it is not possible to differentiate between these
conditions on the basis of the ultrasound findings alone.

Reactive enlargement of lymph nodes can arise in response to a localised inflammatory lesion and a similar appearance may also arise as a result of lymphadenitis although in some cases these glands may become more patchy and heterogeneous in appearance. Neoplasia also commonly produces an increase in size of the cervical lymph nodes. Metastatic spread may produce an increase in the size of the lymph nodes within a localised area while multicentric lymphoma can involve all of the nodes in the cervical chain. Although the appearance of neoplastic nodes is very variable, lymphoma commonly causes a generalised reduction in echogenicity.

Cervical masses

Imaging procedure

A region of hair directly over the lesion and extending a short distance beyond the margins is clipped. The mass itself is imaged in a series of planes depending on its size and location to gain information regarding its internal structure. However, it is also important to scan beyond the boundaries of the mass itself and into the surrounding tissue, which will give information about the exact location of the lesion and also its relationship to adjacent structures. It may be necessary to perform a systematic examination to identify normal regional structures in order to rule them out as the origin of the mass and this can be particularly challenging in the presence of a large lesion which is causing marked disruption of the topography of the region. In addition, it is important to ascertain the relationship of the mass to the major structures in the neck including the blood vessels as this will be of significance when planning a surgical approach or an ultrasound-guided biopsy technique. Small masses which are not palpable may also be identified using ultrasound.

Appearance

The appearance of masses arising from the thyroid and parathyroid glands, larynx and regional lymph nodes has already been described. Other causes of cervical masses can include the presence of a foreign body, haematoma, granuloma, abscess, cellulitis or tumours arising from any other cervical structure. Therefore, the sonographic appearance of a cervical mass will vary depending on its internal composition and the underlying pathological processes involved.

Cystic or fluid-filled areas within a mass will appear as anechoic regions and it is usually possible to differentiate these from vascular structures by altering the angle of the transducer as has been previously described. Cavitated lesions can arise as a result of haemorrhage or necrosis within the mass, producing central regions of mixed echogenicity ranging from hypoechoic to hyperechoic depending on the cellular content of the accumulated material. Soft tissue regions will produce varying degrees of echogenicity depending on their composition, with regions of fat or fibrous tissue producing hyperechoic images, while cellular regions are moderately echogenic and well vascularised or acutely inflamed areas are relatively hypoechoic due to their increased fluid content. Mineralisation within a mass will produce a hyperechoic appearance with distal acoustic shadowing. Masses with a fibrous capsule will have a thin hyperechoic line around their periphery which is visible in any region where the beam is at right angles to the capsule, while masses which are more diffuse or are extending to involve localised structures will have poorly defined margins. These include inflammatory conditions, such as cellulitis, in addition to neoplasia. It is important to assess the extent of these lesions as they may track along between fascial planes (Figure 12.9).

Abscesses commonly consist of a well defined rim of echogenic material with an irregular internal margin, and a central region, which may initially contain swirling echogenic particles representing pus and cell debris or echogenic strands of fibrous tissue. The central area may become progressively more anechoic as the debris sediments out or more echogenic as the pus inspissates. The external margin is also poorly defined and commonly involves adjacent tissue, possibly spreading along between fascial planes although in some instances, it may be localised within well defined external margins. Cellulitis has very poorly defined margins and can extend to involve large regions of the neck but also may produce a hyperechoic rim with a central hypoechoic region. Granulomas appear as complex masses of mixed echogenicity which reflects their composition, including a mixture of fibrous tissue and inflammatory fluid. The appearance of neoplastic masses will also reflect their tissue composition and they are commonly also complex structures of mixed echogenicity. Acute haematomas produce a

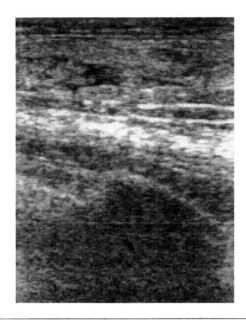

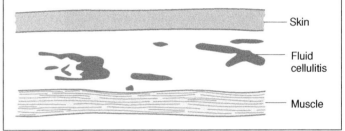

Figure 12.9 Cellulitis in a dog. There is an area of disorganised echogenic material interspersed with irregularly shaped, hypoechoic, fluid-filled regions immediately under the skin surface. The subcutaneous tissue is increased in thickness.

heterogenous echogenic appearance due to the accumulation of red blood cells and will be well marginated if the blood is confined by adjacent structures, although it will be more diffuse with poorly defined margins if it is extending along between the fascial planes of the neck. The appearance will alter as the haematoma resolves, becoming more hypoechoic as the red cells settle out and then more echogenic as the fluid is reabsorbed. A fibrinous network develops producing echogenic strands as the clot resolves.

Lipoma have a characteristic appearance on ultrasound. They have a hypoechoic background superimposed with a series of hyperechoic dots and streaks. They have well defined, smooth, hyperechoic margins and are usually located between structures or within fascial planes (Figure 12.10).

Many lesions which may occur within the cervical region have a similar sonographic appearance and it is not therefore

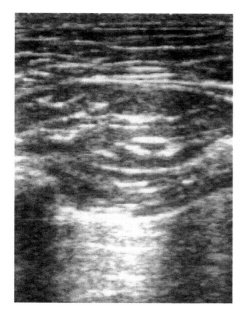

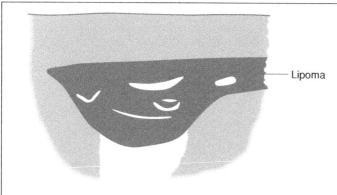

Lipoma

Figure 12.10 Lipoma in the neck. The lipoma is seen here with the characteristic appearance of a hypoechoic background with echogenic streaks throughout. The edges are smooth and well defined and this mass is seen to sit between fascial planes.

possible to differentiate the underlying cause from the ultrasound findings alone. It does help to localise a lesion and determine the extent of local involvement when planning a surgical approach. Ultrasound-guided biopsy or fine-needle aspirate may be indicated in order to reach a diagnosis.

Suggested reading

Bray, J. P., Lipscombe, V. J., White, R. A. S. & Rudorf, H. (1998) Ultra-sonographic Examination of the Pharynx and Larynx of the Normal Dog. In: *Veterinary Radiology and Ultrasound*, **39**, pp. 566–571.

Rudorf, H. & Brown, P. (1998) Ultrasonography of Laryngeal Masses in Six Cats and One Dog. In: *Veterinary Radiology and Ultrasound*, **39**, pp. 430–434.

Sueda, M. T. & Stefanacci, J. D. (2000) Ultrasound Evaluation of the Parathyroid Glands in Two Hypercalcaemic Cats. In: *Veterinary Radiology and Ultrasound*, **41**, pp. 448–451.

Wisner, E. R., Mattoon, J. S., Nyland, T. G. & Baker, T. W. (1991) Normal Ultrasonographic Anatomy of the Canine Neck. In: *Veterinary Radiology and Ultrasound*, **32**, pp. 185–190.

Wisner, E. R. & Nyland, T. G. (1998) Ultrasonography of the Thyroid and Parathyroid Glands. In: *Veterinary Clinics of North America: Small Animal Practice*, **28**:4, pp. 973–991.

Wisner, E. R., Nyland, T. G., Feldman, E. C., *et al.* (1993) Ultrasonographic Evaluation of the Parathyroid Glands in Hypercalcaemic Dogs. In: *Veterinary Radiology and Ultrasound*, **34**, pp. 108–111.

Wisner, E. R., Nyland, T. G. & Mattoon, J. S. (1994) Ultrasonographic Examination of Cervical Masses in the Dog and Cat. In: *Veterinary Radiology and Ultrasound*, **35**, pp. 310–315.

Wisner, E. R., Pennink, D., Biller, D. S., *et al.* (1997) High Resolution Parathyroid Sonography. In: *Veterinary Radiology and Ultrasound*, **38**, pp. 462–466.

Wisner, E. R., Theon, A. P. Thomas, M. S., *et al.* (1994) Ultrasonographic Examination of the Thyroid Gland of Hyperthyroid Cats: Comparison to 99 mTcO-4 Scintigraphy. In: *Veterinary Radiology and Ultrasound*, **35**, pp. 53–58.

Chapter 13

Imaging of the Musculoskeletal System

Alison Dickie

Imaging procedure

Radiography and ultrasound are complementary diagnostic imaging techniques and both have an important role to play in the investigation of the musculoskeletal system. Radiography provides information regarding the configuration and internal structure of the skeleton and also the bony components of joints, due to its ability to penetrate mineralised material. However, as it cannot differentiate well between the soft tissue components of the musculoskeletal system, ultrasound is much better suited to the investigation of these structures. Although initially musculoskeletal ultrasound can appear confusing, with experience and knowledge of regional anatomy, familiarity with the required scan planes will be achieved. This will not only improve the quality of the images produced but also the confidence with which they can be interpreted.

Sonographic examination of the musculoskeletal system is usually performed with the patient in lateral recumbency and the region of interest uppermost, although the animal may be restrained in any comfortable position which allows adequate access to the site. Ensuring the animal is comfortable prior to commencing the scan reduces the likelihood of patient movement and facilitates a systematic, repeatable examination of the area. However, if the region is painful or if the patient is fractious, sedation may be required.

Most musculoskeletal structures are relatively superficial so a high frequency transducer such as 7.5–13 MHz may be used, which ensures that the resulting images are of good resolution. Very superficial structures are best imaged with an echolucent stand-off pad placed between the transducer and the skin surface. The large area of skin surface overlying most regions means that linear or curvilinear transducers can be used. These provide images with excellent near-field definition allowing even very superficial structures to be adequately imaged and so are the transducers of choice. The acoustic window used to examine structures such as the joints is relatively small and this may reduce the quality of an image obtained using a linear transducer as it is not possible to achieve good contact between the skin and the probe. In these cases, microconvex or even sector transducers may be more appropriate although a stand-off pad should be used as near-field distortion occurs with these probes.

Since the ultrasound beam will not penetrate bone, only structures between the bone surface and the transducer can be imaged, this means that the area must be examined from a location where there is no intervening bone. Hair is clipped directly over the region to be scanned, following which surgical spirit then ultrasound coupling gel are applied to the skin surface as elsewhere.

Although ultrasound can distinguish between most components of the musculoskeletal system, the images obtained are often confusing and accurate interpretation relies on the skill and knowledge of the sonographer. It is therefore useful to gain some familiarity with the anatomy of the region under examination by consulting anatomy texts prior to commencing the scan. Most musculoskeletal structures are paired and so it may be beneficial to image the contralateral side of the body allowing comparison between normal and abnormal structures. In many cases this will increase the confidence with which abnormalities can be identified. Each structure should be imaged in the longitudinal plane with the transducer orientated parallel to the long axis of the structure and then in the transverse plane by rotating the transducer through 90° so it is at right angles to the structure. Imaging from a variety of angles is desirable to ensure the entire structure is examined, although in some instances these non-standard images may be difficult to interpret. It is also useful to manipulate the limb during the course of the examination to assess dynamic function as well as static components. Joint instability and tendon ruptures may be identified and larger areas of articular surfaces may be examined.

There is little information available regarding the use of ultrasound to image the musculoskeletal system in the cat rather than the dog, this also reflects the smaller incidence of musculoskeletal disorders encountered in the cat. However, the anatomical structures are sufficiently similar between the species to allow the same approach, although the smaller size and fractious nature of cats may lead to some difficulties.

Bone

Normal appearance

Bone is highly reflective to the ultrasound beam and returns 50% of the beam back to the transducer with the remaining 50% absorbed within the dense material. This results in the production of a hyperechoic line on the image with a strong distal acoustic shadow. The shape of the line will reflect the shape of the soft tissue–bone interface and should be smooth. Only information about the surface of the bone adjacent to the transducer is obtained since the beam does not penetrate any distance into it.

Appearance of abnormalities

Radiography is potentially more useful for investigating bone lesions than ultrasound as it produces information about the internal structure of the bone rather than just the surface. However, ultrasound can be useful to monitor fracture repair in situations where radiography may not be available or metallic implants obscure the region of interest, in addition to allowing assessment and monitoring of adjacent soft tissue involvement.

Any reaction within the periosteum such as that caused by trauma, ligament or tendon damage or degenerative joint disease will produce a roughened contour to the hyperechoic bone interface due to the presence of new bone formation. Inflammatory conditions such as osteomyelitis may also produce roughening of the adjacent bone surface although this is usually also accompanied by heterogeneous, hypoechoic regions within the surrounding soft tissue. An avulsion or chip fracture may be identified as an irregularly shaped hyperechoic structure of variable size embedded in the adjacent soft tissue which produces marked distal acoustic shadowing indicating that it is a mineralised fragment (Figure 13.1). The site of origin may be identified as an irregular defect of comparable size and shape to the fragment in the normally smooth surface of the adjacent bone although this may be obscured by shadowing from the fragment itself, if minimal displacement has occurred.

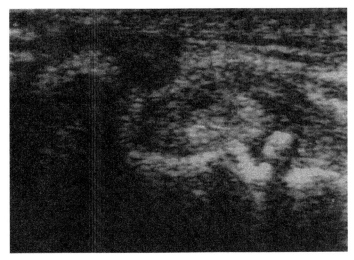

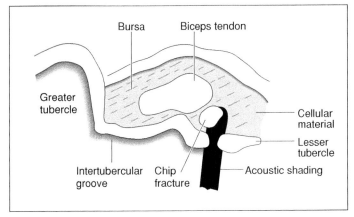

Figure 13.1 Bicipital bursitis and chip fracture of the lesser tubercle of the humerus. The bicipital bursa surrounding the biceps tendon is distended with echogenic material due to the presence of cellular debris. The fracture fragment is visible as a well defined, hyperechoic structure embedded within the adjacent soft tissue and is producing distal acoustic shadowing which indicates that it is mineralised.

A fracture line will often be visible as a discontinuity in the hyperechoic line of the cortex with some transmission of the beam through into the medullary cavity between the two fragments. A step between the two interfaces suggests displacement of one of the fragments. The surrounding area can be examined to determine the extent of any concurrent soft tissue damage such as muscle rupture or haematomas. As healing commences, soft tissue callus appears as a mottled, irregular, poorly marginated, relatively hypoechoic area developing in the region adjacent to the fracture site and will progressively increase in echogenicity with the development of hyperechoic foci producing distal acoustic shadowing as mineralisation progresses. These foci will coalesce until, eventually, the fracture site is obscured and the bony callus is visualised as an irregularly shaped region with a roughened margin and distal acoustic shadowing which will reduce in size and become increasingly smoothly marginated over time.

Metallic implants are very reflective to the beam, and like bone, will produce a well defined hyperechoic line representing the surface of the implant nearest the transducer. In addition to distal acoustic shadowing, reverberation artefacts are also produced due to internal reflections within the implant and appear as 'comet tails' beyond the interface. The beam cannot penetrate through the implant and so the area of bone immediately below is obscured, although the rest of the bone surface can be visualised using a variety of different imaging planes.

Although bone tumours are most commonly investigated using radiography, ultrasound can be useful to determine the degree of invasion into the adjacent soft tissues. The underlying bone surface is commonly markedly disrupted, irregular and roughened although it will remain smooth if the lesion has not yet extended out through the cortex. Mineralised material may be visualised extending out into the adjacent soft tissue where it appears as hyperechoic regions producing distal acoustic shadowing, separate fragments may also be visualised (Figure 13.2). Demineralisation of areas within the lesion or disruption of the cortex will allow penetration of the ultrasound beam and therefore imaging of the internal structure in that region. Ultrasound can be used to guide fine-needle aspirate techniques of the lesions which, if they yield a result, can alleviate the need for the performance of a core biopsy.

Tendons and ligaments

Normal appearance

Tendons have a large fibrous component and therefore contain a large number of tissue interfaces which produce a relatively hyperechoic appearance without distal acoustic shadowing. If the transducer is positioned parallel to the long axis of the tendon, it appears rectangular in shape and the linear arrangement of the tendon fibres can be visualised surrounded by the hyperechoic peritendon (Figure 13.3). The tendon appears most echogenic and the pattern of the fibres can best be appreciated when the beam is at right angles to the tendon. If the transducer is then rotated through

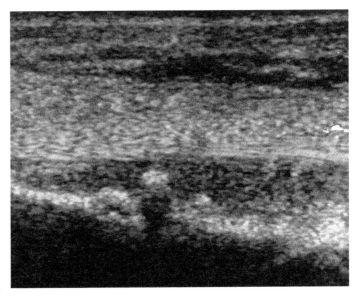

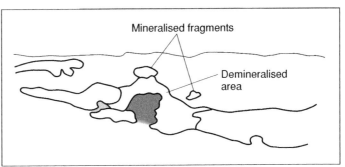

Figure 13.2
Osteosarcoma of the proximal humerus. This is a long-axis view and the underlying bone surface is markedly disrupted and roughened indicating that the tumour has extended out through the cortex. There are also some small, irregularly shaped mineralised fragments within the adjacent soft tissue.

90°, the tendon appears round or oval-shaped in outline, with a regular stippled pattern throughout the body of the tendon, as the fibres are imaged in transverse section and the hyperechoic peritendon is again visualised around the periphery. In some areas the tendon will be surrounded by a tendon sheath which appears as a thin hyperechoic line separated from the tendon by an anechoic region representing the fluid within the sheath. The distance between the sheath and the tendon will therefore depend on the volume of fluid present (Figure 13.4).

The tendon of origin of the biceps brachii muscle arises from the supraglenoid tubercle of the scapula. The tendon crosses the craniomedial aspect of the shoulder joint and runs through the intertubercular groove which is formed between the greater and lesser tubercles of the humerus. This forms a hyperechoic trough when imaged in transverse

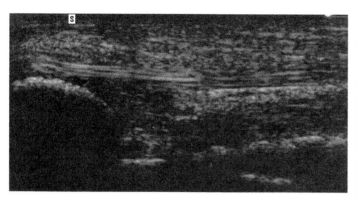

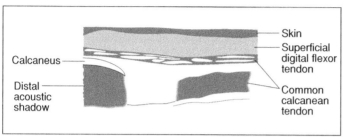

Calcaneus

Distal
acoustic
shadow

Skin
Superficial
digital flexor
tendon

Common
calcanean
tendon

Figure 13.3 Normal calcanean tendon. This is a long-axis view so the tendon appears rectangular and the linear arrangement of the tendon fibres can be visualised. The calcaneus appears as a smooth, slightly convex, hyperechoic line with distal acoustic shadowing and the superficial digital flexor tendon can be visualised as a hyperechoic band running across the calcaneus between it and the skin. Deep to this are the two components of the common calcanean tendon.

section and can be used as an anatomical landmark to identify the biceps tendon which is visualised as an oval-shaped hyperechoic structure within it (Figure 13.4). It is held in place by the transverse humeral retinaculum, a fibrous band running between the greater and lesser tubercles of the humerus, and visualised as a transversely orientated hyperechoic structure. The capsule of the shoulder joint extends into the intertubercular groove and surrounds the tendon to produce the bicipital bursa. This appears as an anechoic region around the periphery of the tendon located between it and the bone surface and the transverse humeral retinaculum. When imaged in long axis, the linear, hyperechoic fibres of the tendon can be seen to arise from the hyperechoic interface of the supraglenoid tubercle and to merge with the muscle belly of the biceps brachii distally.

The tendon of the supraspinatous muscle crosses the cranial aspect of the shoulder joint and can be imaged inserting on to the greater tubercle in a position lateral to the biceps tendon. The supraspinatus and teres minor muscle tendons cross the caudolateral aspect of the joint to insert on to the caudal aspect of the greater tubercle and the teres minor tuberosity respectively.

The common calcanean tendon has contributions from several muscle groups including the gastrocnemius muscle

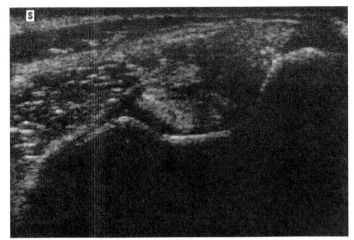

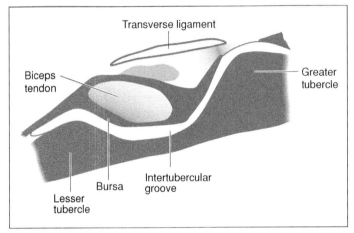

Figure 13.4 Normal tendon of insertion of the biceps brachii muscle. This is a short-axis view so the tendon is an oval-shaped, hyperechoic structure sitting in the hyperechoic trough of the intertubercular groove formed between the greater and lesser tubercles of the humerus. It is held in place by the transverse retinaculum and there is a small volume of fluid which appears as an anechoic region around the tendon between it and the tendon sheath.

located on the caudal aspect of the stifle and tibia and the biceps femoris, semitendinosus and gracilis muscles, which arise from further proximally in the limb. These fuse to form the main two components of the tendon before inserting on to the proximal aspect of the calcaneus where the common calcanean tendon terminates. The superficial digital flexor tendon is located caudally and passes over the caudal aspect of the calcaneus immediately below the skin surface before continuing distally into the pes.

The proximal caudal aspect of the calcaneus appears as a smooth, slightly convex, hyperechoic line with distal acoustic shadowing when imaged in long axis. The superficial digital flexor tendon can be visualised as a hyperechoic band running across the calcaneus between it and the skin surface as it continues distally (Figure 13.3). The component of the common calcanean tendon arising from the medial head of the gastrocnemius can be visualised immediately deep to the superficial digital flexor tendon as a narrow, hyperechoic band with a prominent linear, fibrous pattern. It can be followed to the caudal proximal aspect of the calcaneus where it inserts and is separated from the superficial digital flexor tendon at this point by a bursa. The section of the common calcanean tendon formed from the remaining components is visualised deep to this and is followed distally towards the calcaneus. It inserts on to the medial aspect of the proximal calcaneus and so the angle of the transducer must be altered in order to visualise its point of insertion. There is a second bursa between these two components of the common calcanean tendon.

The long digital extensor tendon can be imaged running from the lateral femoral condyle across the lateral aspect of the stifle joint. The origin of popliteus longus may be imaged between the lateral meniscus where it arises and the joint capsule.

Ligaments also contain a large amount of fibrous tissue and therefore they too appear hyperechoic on ultrasound examination with a linear pattern of parallel fibres. However, in small animals these are mostly small structures and their close association with adjacent soft tissue structures, such as the joint capsule, makes them difficult to differentiate and image as individual structures. The most important exception is the patellar ligament, which is imaged as a linear, hyperechoic structure with well defined hyperechoic margins and central, parallel, linear echoes running across the cranial aspect of the stifle joint from the distal aspect of the patella to insert on to the tibial crest (Figure 13.5).

Appearance of abnormalities

The region of a tendon rupture is usually identifiable due to a complete loss of the normal tendon pattern. The separated, diverging ends of the tendons may be visible proximal and distal to the site and the intervening area will be anechoic or hypoechoic representing the development of a haematoma. Manipulation of the limb may help to identify the two separate ends of the structure. If the rupture has occurred at the point of insertion of the tendon on to bone, then small mineralised bone fragments may be

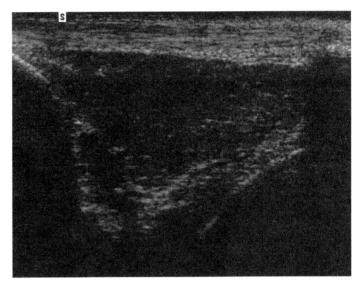

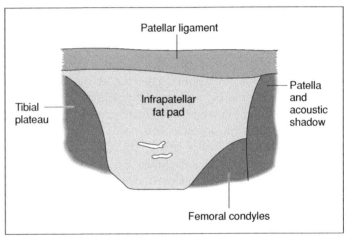

Figure 13.5 Normal stifle joint imaged from the cranial aspect. The patellar ligament is visible as a hyperechoic structure with parallel, linear echoes running across the image from the distal aspect of the patella to insert on to the tibial crest. The curved hyperechoic lines produced by the femoral condyles and tibial plateau form a V-shaped trough deep to the patellar ligament which is filled with an irregular, poorly defined, mottled structure representing the infrapatellar fat pad.

visible in the ends of the tendon and surrounding area as hyperechoic foci which, if of sufficient size, will produce distal acoustic shadowing. Partial rupture results in a region within the tendon where areas of normal tendon pattern will be interspersed with regions of disorganised hypoechoic material and a reduction in the normal linear fibre alignment. This is also usually associated with a localised increase in the diameter of the tendon. Ligamentous damage such as rupture of the patellar ligament will result in a similar sonographic appearance.

As healing of the tendon commences, there will be a gradual increase in echogenicity in these regions representing a reduction in inflammatory fluid and resolution of the haematoma. Fibrous scar tissue is produced within the tendon which increases the echogenicity further, although it is irregular and disorganised lacking the regular linear pattern of the adjacent normal tendon. With time, the diameter of the tendon may reduce and there may be a resolution of the linear pattern, although it may never completely return to normal.

Damage to a tendon may result in an increased accumulation of fluid in the adjacent tendon sheath but this can also arise as a result of localised inflammation or infection. This fluid is easily recognised as an anechoic region surrounding the tendon, the size of which will vary with the volume of fluid. Any cellular debris or haemorrhage within this fluid will result in a hypoechoic or echogenic appearance (Figure 13.1, p. 254). Tendinitis will result in irregular, hypoechoic, mottled regions within the tendon due to the accumulation of inflammatory fluid and a loss of distinction in the fibre pattern of the adjacent areas (Figure 13.6). In chronic cases, the tendon may become increased in thickness with patchy hypoechoic and also hyperechoic areas representing the accumulation of cells or scar tissue. Deposition of calcium may also occur producing hyperechoic foci which will demonstrate distal acoustic shadowing if of sufficient size. Calcification of the supraspinatus tendon may also occur and will have a similar appearance (Figure 13.7).

It is possible for the tendon of origin of the biceps brachii to become dislocated from the intertubercular groove following rupture of the transverse ligament. This results in the identification of an empty groove when imaging in short axis although in some cases the tendon may be located in the region of the lesser tubercle.

Although the individual ligamentous structures associated with a joint cannot be differentiated from adjacent soft tissue structures, damage to the ligament will result in the formation of a haematoma which is readily visualised as a hypoechoic region.

Joints

Imaging procedure

The shoulder and coxofemoral joints are surrounded by a large number of soft tissue structures resulting in a limited

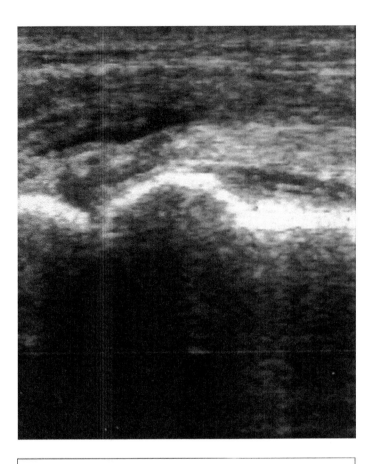

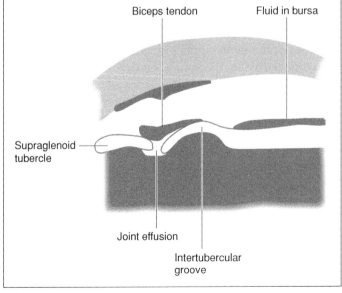

Figure 13.6 Biciptal tenosynovitis. There is distension of the bicipital bursa and the shoulder joint space. The tendon of origin of the biceps is irregular in outline and mottled with hypoechoic and hyperechoic patches representing inflammation and disruption of the fibre pattern.

Biceps tendon

Fluid in bursa

Supraglenoid tubercle

Joint effusion

Intertubercular groove

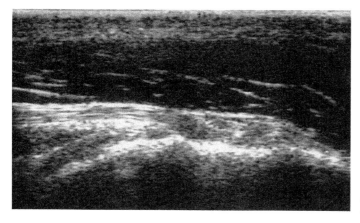

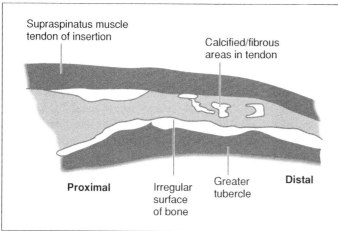

Supraspinatus muscle tendon of insertion

Calcified/fibrous areas in tendon

Proximal

Irregular surface of bone

Greater tubercle

Distal

Figure 13.7
Calcification of the tendon of insertion of the supraspinatus muscle. Disruption of the fibre pattern results in a mottled appearance to the tendon with the calcium deposits producing hyperechoic areas, which will demonstrate distal acoustic shadowing if of sufficient size. The underlying bone surface appears irregular and roughened suggesting the presence of new bone formation.

number of areas where the transducer can be placed in order to obtain adequate images. Further distally the joints have less intervening soft tissue but their small size means that the acoustic windows available for imaging the joint space itself are limited. In addition, deeper structures may not be visualised if there is intervening bone or they are located beyond the depth to which the high frequency beam can easily penetrate. Therefore it is not always possible to image the entire articular surface of a joint. However, once the joint space has been located, manipulation will usually allow most of the clinically relevant areas to be visualised and so ultrasound is a useful technique in the investigation of joint abnormalities. This will also permit a dynamic evaluation of joint function to identify the presence of instability or abnormal movement. However, if the joint is painful then sedation may be required to allow an adequate examination of the joint to be performed.

The shoulder joint is best imaged from the lateral aspect with the transducer applied distal to the acromion process of the scapular spine. Manipulation will allow most of the caudal aspect of the head of the humerus to be examined. It is not possible to examine this joint from the caudal or medial aspects due to the close apposition of the proximal limb to the body and the cranial acoustic window is limited by the greater tubercle of the humerus.

The hip joint can be imaged from the ventral aspect by positioning the patient in dorsal recumbency and applying the transducer to the skin surface directly over the coxofemoral joint. It can also be imaged from the dorsal surface with the animal standing or in lateral recumbency and the transducer angled between the greater trochanter and the ischium. Again, manipulation may be useful to assess joint function.

The remaining joints in the limb have fewer soft tissue structures around them and so they are imaged by placing the transducer directly over the region of interest. Their superficial nature means that the use of a stand-off pad between the transducer and the skin surface may be necessary to allow adequate imaging.

Due to the complex nature of the stifle joint, a series of different approaches has been recommended to ensure that all of the important structures are imaged. From the cranial aspect the transducer can be applied distal and then proximal to the patella in both vertical and horizontal positions. Imaging can also be performed from the medial and lateral aspects, although from these positions sagittal images are most useful since horizontal ones are difficult to interpret. It is more difficult to image the stifle from a caudal approach due to the large muscle mass in this region which limits access and increases the distance between the transducer and the joint resulting in images of poor quality. In all locations, the joint should be manipulated and examined in flexion and extension.

Normal appearance

Joint spaces themselves are narrow and are located between the adjacent bone surfaces which appear as smooth, curved, hyperechoic lines producing distal acoustic shadowing.

The shape of these corresponds closely with each other and reflects the shape of the epiphyses. Cartilage has a high water content and therefore appears almost anechoic on the ultrasound image as it does not produce much attenuation of the beam. It is visible as a dark line adjacent to and matching the shape of the underlying subchondral bone and should be of even thickness. The anechoic joint fluid is located between the surfaces of the articular cartilage but the volume is usually too small to be easily appreciable. The joint capsule may be visible at the periphery of the joint space as a thin hyperechoic line, which merges with the structures surrounding the joint. In joints such as the stifle, the collateral ligaments and the joint capsule cannot be differentiated using ultrasound.

In young puppies, the femoral head appears as a hyperechoic spherical structure sitting within the hyperechoic circle representing the acetabulum. The centre of ossification within the femoral head produces a hyperechoic focus which increases in size as calcification progresses and after approximately eight weeks of age there is a sufficient distal acoustic shadowing to obscure the articular surface of the acetabulum located deep to it. Following this, only the edge of the acetabulum and the surface of the femoral head closest to the transducer are visible. The joint capsule is visible as a thin, convex, echogenic line running between the margins of the acetabulum and peripheral to the femoral head.

When imaging the stifle in long axis from the cranial aspect distal to the patella, the patellar ligament is visible as a linear, hyperechoic structure with well defined hyperechoic margins and central, parallel, linear echoes. It extends across the image from the distal aspect of the patella to insert on to the tibial crest (Figure 13.5, p. 260). If a stand-off pad is used, the skin and underlying fascia appear as a homogenous, moderately echogenic layer located between the patellar ligament and the transducer. The patella appears as a curved hyperechoic line with distal acoustic shadowing. The curved hyperechoic lines produced by the femoral condyles and tibial plateau form a V-shaped trough deep to the patellar ligament which is filled with an irregular, poorly defined, mottled structure representing the infrapatellar fat pad. Flexion of the joint and rotation of the transducer may allow the cranial regions of the cruciate ligaments to be identified. These appear hypoechoic relative to the surrounding fat although the more caudal regions of these structures are not visible due to the shape of the joint. The cranial cruciate is visualised where it attaches to the cranial intercondylar area of the tibia and then runs to between the femoral condyles while the caudal cruciate may be imaged attaching to the lateral surface of the medial femoral condyle.

Proximal to the patella, the junction between the hyperechoic patellar ligament and the hypoechoic quadriceps femoris muscle can be evaluated. The proximal extremity of the stifle joint space is visualised as an anechoic region proximal to the patella between the shaft of the femur and the quadriceps. When imaged in short axis, the patellar ligament becomes oval-shaped in outline and moving the transducer proximally allows the trochlear ridges and patellar groove of the distal femur to be visualised as a smooth, M-shaped, hyperechoic line. The patella should be imaged located within this groove.

Imaging in a sagittal plane from the lateral and medial aspect of the stifle allows the peripheral regions of the meniscii to be visualised as homogenous, echogenic, triangular-shaped structures tapering into the V-shaped joint space formed between the tibial plateau and the femoral condyles (Figure 13.8). The base of the menisci is confluent

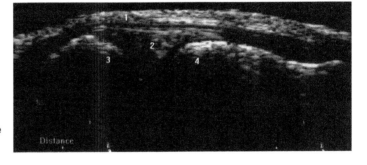

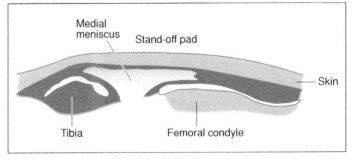

Figure 13.8 Normal stifle imaged from the medial aspect. The peripheral region of the medial meniscus appears as a homogenous, echogenic, triangular-shaped structure tapering into the V-shaped joint space formed between the tibial plateau and the femoral condyles. It is not possible to distinguish the medial collateral ligaments from the overlying joint capsule.

with the joint capsule. The caudal approach only allows visualisation of the caudal musculature of the limb and a small area of the caudal aspect of the joint space and femoral condyles but does not allow visualisation of the caudal cruciate ligament.

Appearance of abnormalities

Ultrasound is particularly useful in the investigation of swollen joints as it can differentiate between joint effusions and swelling of the surrounding soft tissue. An increased volume of fluid within a joint space will result in an anechoic region extending beyond the normal margins of the joint the size of which will vary depending on the volume of fluid present. This may cause distension and distortion of the surrounding synovial membrane making it easier to identify. It may enhance the appearance of the surrounding structures, especially if it extends into a tendon bursa which communicates with the joint space, although it can also result in the displacement of adjacent structures such as the infrapatellar fat pad of the stifle. The hypoechoic layer of articular cartilage may appear to be separated from the fluid by an echogenic margin which represents the interface between the two substances. Any cellular debris or haemorrhage within the fluid will result in an increased echogenicity ranging from hypoechoic to echogenic.

Thickening of the joint capsule can also occur and results in the normally thin hyperechoic structure becoming a broad band with indistinct margins. Many conditions affecting joints will result in peri-articular new bone formation and this will produce a roughened, irregular contour to the hyperechoic bone interface. Tumours arising within the joint will have a variable appearance depending on the tissue type present but will usually be identified as irregularly shaped, poorly margined structures of mixed echogenicity occupying the joint space. They may extend into the adjacent soft tissue causing marked disruption of the local anatomy and may also involve the underlying bone producing roughened areas with defects in the hyperechoic margins if the cortex has been breached. Ultrasound can also differentiate between joint effusions and hygromas, which are fluid-filled regions over bony protruberances such as the olecranon and calcaneus and do not involve underlying joint space or bursae.

Manipulation of a joint during the examination may reveal the presence of instability or subluxation as identified by an increased distance or abnormal motion of the components of the joint relative to each other. Complete luxation will result in an empty or absent joint space depending on the joint under investigation and the displaced bony components may be identified embedded within the surrounding soft tissue. The accumulation of fibrin within the joint space in chronic cases may be identified as an irregular, mottled region of material ranging from hypoechoic to hyperechoic in appearance. Ultrasound can also be useful for assessing the extent of the resulting damage caused to the surrounding soft tissue structures.

Osteochondrosis lesions may be visualised on the articular surface of the humeral head or femoral condyles. In these regions, the hypoechoic layer of articular cartilage is disrupted and the smooth curved hyperechoic surface of the underlying subchondral bone may also demonstrate a defect of varying size and shape producing a roughened area. Separate osteochondrosis dissecans fragments may be visualised adjacent to the defect or at various locations within the joint space as hyperechoic structures and they may also produce distal acoustic shadowing if they are mineralised. In the shoulder joint they may migrate craniodistally where they can be imaged as hyperechoic structures located in the bicipital bursa between the biceps tendon and the bone surface of the intertubercular groove.

Avascular necrosis of the femoral head may be identified using ultrasound if the resulting demineralisation allows the ultrasound beam to penetrate beyond the bone surface. The hyperechoic surface of the bone will be roughened and irregular and the amount of distal acoustic shadowing it produces will be reduced resulting in echoes being returned from the internal structure. Widening of the joint space may result in visualisation of a section of the articular surface of the acetabulum.

Damage such as tearing of the menisci of the stifle can sometimes be identified with careful examination as echogenic lines running across these normally homogenous structures. They may also become detached from the joint capsule although this may be easier to appreciate in the presence of a joint effusion. Chronic degenerative changes within the menisci may result in them appearing mottled and irregular. It is not usually possible to identify the cranial cruciate ligament if it has acutely ruptured, although with chronicity, the ends of the structure appear hyperechoic and therefore become easier to visualise.

Muscle

Normal appearance

Muscle is very vascular and therefore appears hypoechoic on the ultrasound image. However, the fibrous tissue surrounding each of the muscle bundles within it produces a series of hyperechoic lines throughout the muscle belly. This creates a coarse, striated appearance when the muscle is imaged in long axis and a more reticular pattern of scattered echoes in short axis (Figure 13.9). The sonographic appearance of muscle will therefore vary depending on the angle at which it is imaged although the pattern also varies between different muscles according to the orientation of the bundles. In addition, each muscle is surrounded by connective tissue fascia which produces a well defined, smooth, hyperechoic margin allowing differentiation from adjacent muscle groups. During contraction, the thickness of the muscular body will increase and therefore the dimensions of each muscle are not constant.

Appearance of abnormalities

Space occupying lesions may be identified within muscular tissue including seroma, haematoma, abscess or tumour formation. Ultrasound can provide information regarding the size and margination of the region and its extension into the adjacent muscle tissue or other surrounding structures. Lesions confined within the muscle belly itself tend to be round or oval in shape and surrounded by a margin of muscle tissue. However, those located outside the muscle will have a more variable outline and may appear elongated or spindle-shaped as they conform to the outline of adjacent structures and track along fascial planes following the path of least resistance. Information regarding its internal structure may help to reach a tentative diagnosis such as in the case of seroma, which appears as an accumulation of anechoic fluid.

Abscesses commonly consist of a well defined rim of echogenic material with an irregular internal margin and a

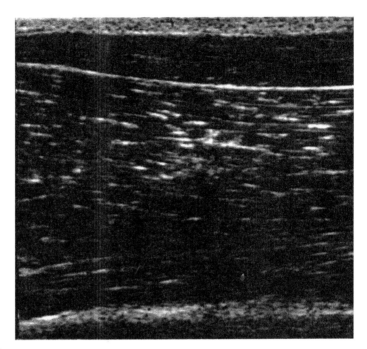

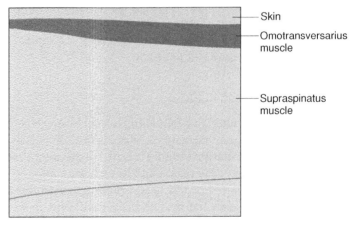

Skin

Omotransversarius muscle

Supraspinatus muscle

Figure 13.9 Normal supraspinatus and omotransversarius muscles. The muscle bellies appear hypoechoic with a series of hyperechoic lines produced by the fibrous tissue throughout, the pattern of which will alter with the imaging plane. The supraspinatus muscle is imaged in long axis and appears to have a coarse, striated appearance while the omotransversarius is imaged in short axis and has a finer, more reticular pattern of scattered echoes. It is therefore easy to differentiate between muscle groups using ultrasound.

central region which may initially contain swirling echogenic particles representing pus and cell debris or echogenic strands of fibrous tissue producing compartmentalisation of the lesion. The central area may become progressively more anechoic as the debris settles out or more echogenic as the pus inspissates. The presence of gas may produce a series of hyperchoic foci with distal reverberation or ring-down artefact, and these may be mobile within the lumen or fixed within the echogenic pus. The external margin is usually poorly defined and commonly involves adjacent tissue, possibly spreading along fascial planes or to involve local joints, although in some instances it may be localised within well defined external margins.

Acute haematomas produce a heterogenous echogenic appearance due to the accumulation of red blood cells and will vary in shape depending on whether the blood has accumulated between or within muscles. Occasionally the vessel from which it has arisen can be imaged in the area. The sonographic appearance will alter as the haematoma resolves, becoming more hypoechoic as the red cells settle out and then more echogenic as the fluid is resorbed. A fibrinous network develops producing echogenic strands as the clot resolves. The sonographic appearance of neoplastic masses will also reflect their tissue composition and therefore they are very variable. It is important to assess the surrounding soft tissue and bony structures for evidence of invasion.

Strain injuries resulting in the tearing of fibres within a muscle and their subsequent healing will follow a similar pattern to that of tendon or ligament damage. There will be an area within the muscle which is increased in thickness, lacks a normal pattern and has an accumulation of hypoechoic inflammatory fluid and haemorrhage. The extent of the changes observed will depend on the severity of the damage incurred right through to complete rupture where manipulation of the limb may help to identify the clubbed ends of the ruptured muscle mass. The muscle bellies will contract away from the rupture and will therefore appear increased in thickness but with an otherwise normal sonographic appearance. In some cases, rather than muscle rupture, avulsion of either the tendon of insertion or origin will occur, resulting in contraction of the muscle belly away from the area of injury.

Recurrent or chronic injuries may result in the production of fibrous scars within the muscle rather than normal healing. These appear as echogenic or hyperechoic bands on ultrasound which do not change in size when the muscle contracts. Calcification may also occur producing hyperechoic regions within the muscle which, if large enough, will produce distal acoustic shadowing. Contractures may occur in the supraspinatus, infraspinatus, quadriceps, semi-membranosus and gracilis muscles and are also associated with regions of echogenic or hyperechoic fibrous tissue.

Disuse atrophy results in a reduction in mass of otherwise normal appearing muscle.

Nerves and blood vessels

Imaging procedure

Good anatomical knowledge is required to image specific peripheral nerves and blood vessels and most commonly they are identified while examining other aspects of the musculoskeletal system.

The brachial plexus is formed from the ventral branches of the spinal nerves from the level of C6 to T2 and is located on the medial aspect of the scapula. An area of hair is clipped on the cranial aspect of the limb proximal and medial to the shoulder joint and the transducer applied.

Normal appearance

Nerves and blood vessels often follow a similar course through the limb and may be identified using local anatomical landmarks as a bundle running between muscle groups. Both have round or oval hyperechoic margins but blood vessels have an anechoic lumen while nerves have a stippled hyperechoic centre. Rotation of the transducer through 90° allows these structures to be imaged in long axis as narrow parallel hyperechoic lines with nerves containing a series of linear internal echoes and blood vessels having an anechoic lumen. It is often difficult to differentiate between small nerves and blood vessels without using Doppler ultrasound to identify the presence or absence of blood flow, although increasing the frequency of the transducer may help in some instances. In some instances, visualisation of pulsation within arteries and compression of veins may be possible.

Appearance of abnormalities

An important application of ultrasound when imaging peripheral vascular structures and nerves is to assess their relationship to nearby lesions. Masses may distort the normal anatomy, resulting in them being displaced and following an abnormal or tortuous route. Alternatively, the lesion may surround them and loss of the well defined hyperechoic outer walls of these structures may suggest that invasion has occurred. The patency of blood vessels should also be assessed as compression may occur as a result of surrounding lesions, and echogenic material may be visualised within the lumen suggesting invasion or thrombus formation has occurred. In some cases, Doppler ultrasound may be required to identify this compromise by demonstrating variances in the blood flow through the vessel. In addition, identification of major blood vessels within, or adjacent to, a lesion will help to plan an approach for ultrasound-guided aspirate or biopsy techniques or a surgical procedure.

Ultrasound can be useful for the identification of brachial plexus tumours (Figure 13.10). These are identified by their anatomical location and appear as round or oval-shaped masses of mixed echogenicity with hypoechoic regions of nervous tissue interspersed with anechoic blood vessels.

Lymph nodes and other superficial structures

Normal appearance

Normal lymph nodes are identified as oval-shaped or fusiform, hypoechoic structures with well defined smooth margins. The popliteal lymph node may be imaged in its location within the fascia, caudal to the stifle joint. However, the other peripheral lymph nodes are not usually identified unless they are enlarged.

Adipose tissue accumulates in the subcutaneous region and also within the fascia surrounding the musculoskeletal system, with the amount present depending on the body condition of the animal and also the region being examined. The large number of interfaces within the adipose tissue produces a patchy appearance with irregular hypoechoic areas interspersed with disorganised hyperechoic linear structures. Its lack of distinct margins and diffuse nature allow it to be easily differentiated from adjacent muscle bellies. Adipose tissue attenuates the ultrasound beam quite markedly resulting in a reduction in the distance that the beam can penetrate. This may be problematic if deeper structures are being examined in a patient with large amounts of subcutaneous adipose tissue.

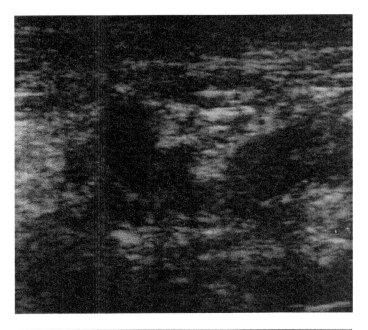

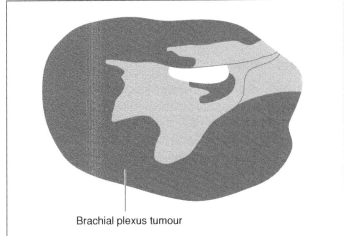

Figure 13.10 Brachial plexus tumour. The tumour is seen as an oval-shaped mass of mixed echogenicity with hypoechoic regions of nervous tissue.

Brachial plexus tumour

Appearance of abnormalities

Ultrasound may help to locate foreign material within either the soft tissues of the limb or the footpad in a three-dimensional plane which is not usually possible using radiography. In acute cases, many foreign bodies contain or are surrounded by air which produces a hyperechoic appearance with distal acoustic shadowing and reverberation

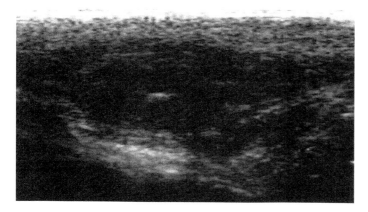

(a)

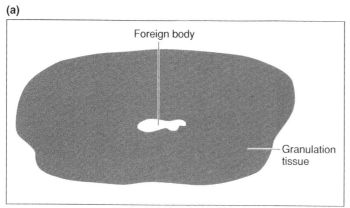

Foreign body

Granulation
tissue

Figure 13.11 a & b
Thorn foreign body in
the submandibular
region of a dog. A
well defined, hypo-
echoic, subcutaneous
nodule containing a
hyperechoic focus,
which represents the
foreign material, can
be seen and this is
surrounded by a
localised hypoechoic
region produced by
granulation tissue and
inflammatory fluid.

artefact. Likewise, metallic objects have a characteristic appearance as they produce reverberation which causes a distinctive ring-down or comet-tail artefact. However, in more chronic cases, a region of granulation tissue accumulates around the site which appears as a hypoechoic zone around the foreign body (Figure 13.11 a & b). Depending on the location of the material, infection may spread along the fascial planes to produce a cellulitis or may be confined to form a localised abscess; the appearance of these conditions has been described in Chapter 12, p. 247. With time, porous objects, such as wood, will absorb fluid, lose their distinctive appearance and may become more difficult to differentiate from the surrounding granulation tissue with its mixed echogenicity.

Ultrasound is also useful for the investigation of masses and this has been described in Chapter 12, p. 246.

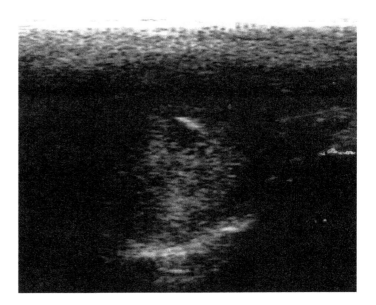

(b)

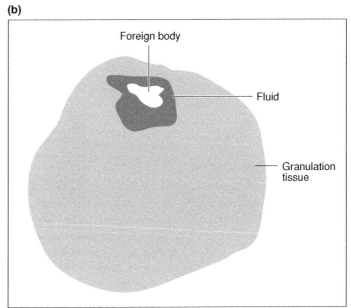

Foreign body

Fluid

Granulation tissue

Figure 13.11 a & b
(*continued*)

Suggested reading

Hudson, J. A., Steiss, J. E., Braund, K. G., *et al.* (1996) Ultrasonography of Peripheral Nerves During Wallerian Degeneration and Regeneration Following Transection. In: *Veterinary Radiology and Ultrasound*, **37**, pp. 302–312.

Kramer, M., Gerwing, M., Hach, V., *et al.* (1997) Sonography of the Musculoskeletal System in Dogs and Cats. In: *Veterinary Radiology and Ultrasound*, **38**, pp. 139–149.

Kramer, M., Stengel, H., Gerwing, M., *et al.* (1999) Sonography of the Canine Stifle. In: *Veterinary Radiology and Ultrasound*, **40**, pp. 282–293.

Long, C. D. & Nyland, T. G. (1999) Ultrasonographic Evaluation of the Canine shoulder. In: *Veterinary Radiology and Ultrasound*, **40**, pp. 372–379.

Reed, A. L., Payne, J. T. & Constantinescu, G. M. (1995) Ultrasonographic Anatomy of the Normal Canine Stifle. In: *Veterinary Radiology and Ultrasound*, **36**, pp. 315–321.

Chapter 14

Imaging of the Eye and Orbit

Val Schmid

Ocular sonography

Imaging procedure

Although A-mode sonography is used for examination of the eye, specialised equipment is required and discussion of this particular technique is beyond the scope of this chapter, which will deal with B-mode and Doppler examinations. There is a number of indications for sonography of the eye and peri-orbital area, including ocular trauma, and to assess the deeper structures of the eye when ophthalmoscopy is precluded. It is also indicated to help classify congenital abnormalities such as persistent hyperplastic tunica vasculosa lentis/persistent hyperplastic primary vitreous (PHTVL/PHPV), to confirm or eliminate ocular or retrobulbar masses and in ocular biometry. While B mode allows assessment of ocular anatomy, colour and power Doppler examinations allow assessment of the vascularity of ocular and orbital masses and help characterise vascular malformations and other vascular diseases. These techniques also allow differentiation of vitreous from retinal detachments.

A 7.5 or 10 MHz transducer with a small contact surface (sector, microconvex or linear probe) is acceptable for ocular examination. The use of a stand-off pad is usually not necessary, except for examination of the anterior segment of the eye. To maximise lateral resolution, the area of interest should fall within the focal zone and a dynamic focussing system is an advantage, since it allows placing the focal zone in the near field or anywhere desired. If the focal zone is fixed, a stand-off pad may be required to achieve this.

The direct corneal contact method is preferred, following application of a topical anaesthetic and enough standard sonographic gel. Scanning through the eyelids and the use of a sterile gel is necessary only in cases where the cornea is damaged, such as trauma or corneal ulceration. After the examination the eye should be rinsed with sterile saline solution.

Various scanning planes are used including axial, trans-scleral, tangential and temporal approaches. For the axial approach, scan along the central optic axis, through the centres of curvature from the vertex of the cornea to the posterior pole, in a transverse and sagittal plane. This is most useful for general screening and orientation. With the transscleral approach, scanning through the lens is avoided, and this is considered best for imaging structures in the posterior segment such as the retina. In the tangential approach (Figure 14.1), the transducer is not perpendicular to the cornea but applied against it. This is used to display anterior structures such as the iris. With the temporal approach, the probe

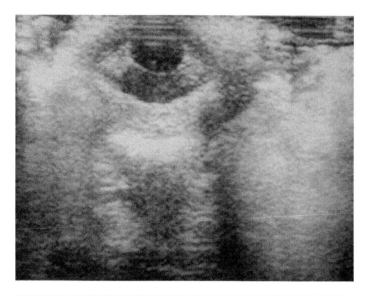

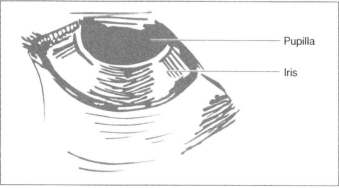

Pupilla

Iris

Figure 14.1
Tangential section of the iris. The iris is seen as a circular grey-shaded area around the central hypoechoic, rounded pupil.

is placed caudal to the orbital ligament and directed ventrally. This is especially useful for orbital scanning and especially for visualisation of the optical nerve and extra-ocular muscles.

Most patients will allow the examination with gentle restraint and topical anaesthesia. Sedation or anaesthesia has the disadvantage that the eye will retract into the orbit and the globe will rotate downwards, making visualisation and orientation difficult.

There are some general screening principles which should be implemented when scanning the eye. A systematic approach is vital, placing the beam perpendicular to the interfaces of interest such as the cornea and lens, as these are specular reflectors. The lowest possible gain should be used to optimise resolution and avoid artefacts. After a general screening examination to allow lesion detection, a topographic examination should be made defining precisely the exact location, extension, shape, echogenicity and echotexture of the lesions. Sensitivity variation techniques can be of some help in differentiating retinal tears from other membranes because the detached retina can be detected at a much lower level of amplification than vitreous membranes. With a 'kinetic exam' we try to observe the mobility of point-like or membranous lesions during and after natural rotation of the globe. This dynamic examination will also help in the differentiation of membranes, although it needs a lot of experience to be interpreted. A detached retina will show a moderate mobility following movement of the globe and a lot of inertia (minimal after-movements), whereas other membranes (e.g. of vitreous origin) show a marked mobility and marked after-movements.

Normal appearance

The normal globe is an anechoic sphere and is divided anatomically into two sonographically visible compartments – the anterior and posterior segments (Figure 14.2). The anterior segment comprises the cornea, the anterior and posterior chambers (potential spaces situated respectively between the posterior surface of the cornea and the anterior surface of the iris, and between the posterior surface of the iris and the anterior lens capsule), the iris, the ciliary body and the lens. The posterior segment (from the periphery to the centre) comprises the sclera, the choroid, the retina, optic disc and vitreous.

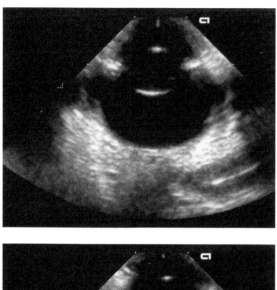

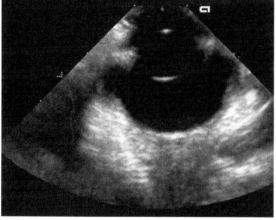

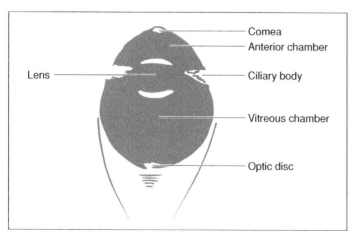

Figure 14.2   Normal eye.

Abnormal appearance

Ocular masses

The first step is to characterise the mass according to location, shape, size, extension, echogenicity and echotexture. The other ocular structures are then assessed. Masses within the globe can be cystic, solid or mixed. Cystic lesions are rare and as such only iridal cysts will be considered. Solid and mixed lesions can be of neoplastic, infectious or inflammatory origin or represent organised haemorrhages. Primary ocular neoplasms are rare in dogs and cats. In the anterior segment the most common neoplasms are of melanocytic origin. They often arise from the iris stroma and spread into the ciliary body and irido-corneal angle (Figure 14.3). Rarely, they may extend posteriorly and involve the choroid or the sclera. In cats these carry a higher rate of metastatic spread and their prognosis is dependent on extension. The

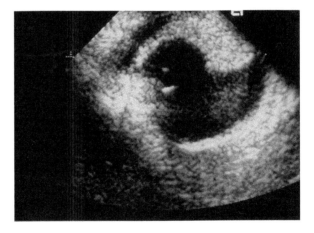

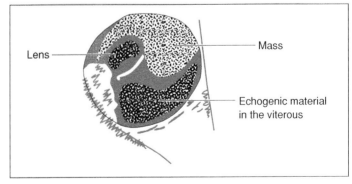

Figure 14.3
Melanoma arising from the iris in a dog. A large homogeneous mass fills the anterior part of the eye. The mass surrounds the lens, which is dislocated medially and in a posterior direction. Echogenic material is visible in the vitreous.

sonographic exam can be a useful tool for this assessment. These masses appear often hyperechoic, with a homogenous parenchyma. Sometimes a diffuse thickening of the whole circumference of the iris will be noted instead of a localised mass. As their size increases they tend to displace the lens. Other ciliary body neoplasms include ciliary body adenomas and adenocarcinomas, and metastatic lesions.

Choroidal masses are rare in dogs and cats. They can be of fungal (most commonly blastomycosis), parasitic or neoplastic origin. The most common metastatic ocular neoplasm is lymphosarcoma, which is also the most common intra-ocular neoplasm. Ocular metastases can theoretically be localised anywhere in the globe and can also be bilateral. The sonographic appearance of metastatic ocular tumours has not been extensively reported in dogs and cats.

Infection (especially oculomycoses), inflammation and organising haemorrhage can also present as intra-ocular mass lesions. They are localised usually in the posterior segment.

A more or less mobile ovoid mass in the posterior ocular segment with a hyperechoic capsule usually represents a luxated lens, especially when the normal specular reflections of the anterior and posterior lens wall are missing.

Ocular membranes

Ocular membranes can originate from retinal detachment, posterior vitreous detachment or other causes such as adhesions, cyclitic membranes and vascular remnants. Remember that a transscleral approach, avoiding the lens, is sometimes useful to visualise these structures.

Membranes not visibly attached to the optic nerve head

Echogenic membranes, inserting abruptly into the globe wall are described in human medicine as being typical of choroidal detachments. These are rare in dogs and cats. Echogenic membranes gradually merging with the globe wall can represent early incomplete retinal detachment.

A linear membrane, where the distance from the posterior ocular wall increases at the upper quadrant (on a vertical axial scan) and which has some areas of adhesions with the underlying retina, is consistent with a posterior vitreous detachment. Demarcation of areas with intravitreal opacities from a clear (anechoic) retro-hyaloid space is another

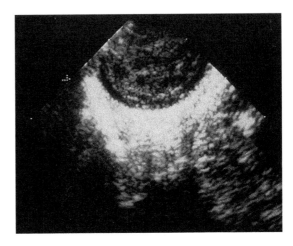

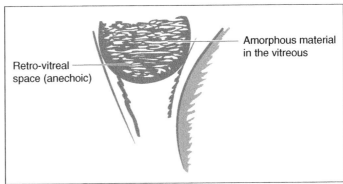

Retro-vitreal
space (anechoic)

Amorphous material
in the vitreous

Figure 14.4
Intravitreal bleeding.
Note the amorphous
opacities in the
vitreous and the clear,
anechoic retrovitreal
space, suggesting
vitreous detachment.

important feature (Figure 14.4). Remember that the vitreous detachment forms a membrane resulting from organisation of haemorrhage or inflammation and this is thinner, less echogenic and more mobile (with after-movements) than retinal or choroidal membranes.

Membranes visibly attached to the optic nerve head

Complete, open-funnel retinal detachments produce a typical V-shaped opacity anchored to the optic nerve head. The angle of the 'V' depends on the degree of vitreo-retinal traction and/or adhesion.

A folded retina or a closed-funnel detachment appears like an echo-dense line running from the optic disc to the posterior lens capsule and represents an old total retinal detachment with secondary proliferative vitreo-retinopathy (Figure 14.5).

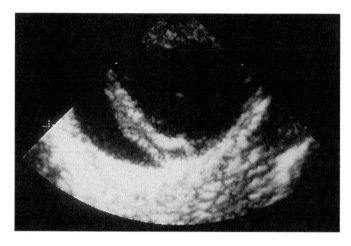

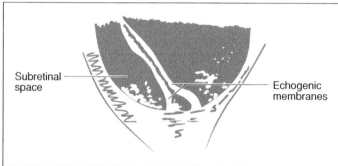

Figure 14.5 Posterior part of the globe of a 12-year-old poodle with retinal detachment. Two echogenic membranes are in close vicinity, probably because they have fused, forming a so-called closed-funnel retinal detachment. They can be followed up to the optic nerve. The subretinal space shows some dispersed opacities.

In long-standing detachments, other membranes (cord opacities) or cysts are visible along the retinal folds or in the subretinal space, producing a very confused appearance. Sometimes a retinal tear will be visible and the edges of the break will be more or less rolled (Figure 14.6 a & b).

Other membranes

Funnel-shaped retrolenticular membranes or tissue opacities attached to the posterior lens capsule coursing along the optic axis to the optic disc can be detected sonographically and represent a congenital condition called persistent hyperplastic primary vitreous/persistent hyperplastic tunica vasculosa lentis (PHPV/PHTVL). Sometimes these membranes will contain a pulsating vessel, visible on 2-D and/or duplex colour or power Doppler examination, representing a persistent hyaloid artery (Figure 14.7 a & b). A persistent hyaloid artery without associated posterior capsular opacities

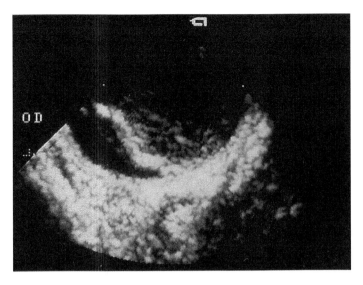

(a)

Figure 14.6 a
Posterior part of the globe of a dog with a cataract and retinal detachment. Note the thick echogenic membrane that can be followed up to the optic nerve. Amorphous opacities are seen in the vitreous.

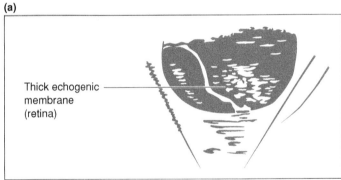

Thick echogenic membrane (retina)

can also be observed and is usually not clinically significant if no other lenticular, vitreal or retinal anomalies are detected.

Ocular opacities

Ocular opacities can be described relative to their location (anterior *vs.* posterior segment, lens), extension and echostructure. The sonographic examination of ocular opacities is mandatory only when these opacities preclude the ophtalmoscopic exam.

Opacities originating from the anterior segment that can hinder the ophtalmoscopic exam include dense corneal opacities, hyphaema (bleeding in the anterior chamber) and hypopyon (accumulation of pus in the anterior chamber). Hyphaema (and less frequently, vitreous haemorrhage) is

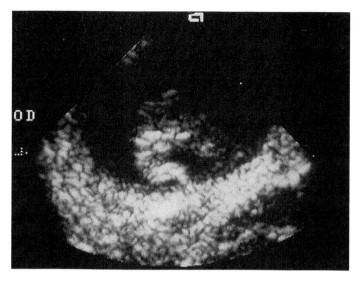

(b)

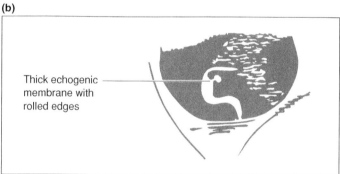

Thick echogenic
membrane with
rolled edges

Figure 14.6 b Same
eye as (a) but using a
different plane. The
thick membrane
shows rolled edges
suggesting a retinal
tear.

occasionally seen in hypertensive cats. These cats are often
presented with sudden blindness secondary to retinopathy.
In these cases the ultrasonographic screening for retinal detachment is indicated. With anterior uveitis and posterior
synechia (iris adhesion with anterior lens capsule), the anterior chamber is echogenic, the iris is thickened and the
anterior lens capsule is irregular. Iris and ciliary body masses
or cysts will also produce opacity in the anterior segment.

Opacities originating from the lens are due to dense cataract formation. The cataract produces abnormal echoes in
the normally anechoic lens. While sonography is not a precise tool in the classification of cataracts, it is recommended
in pre-operative cataract screening to check the retrolenticular
structures for diseases like retinal detachment, vitreous
degeneration or optic disc cupping.

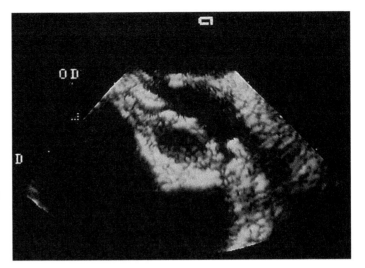

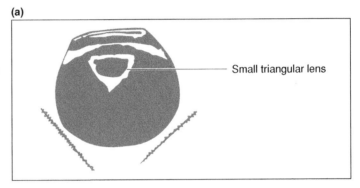

(a)

Small triangular lens

Figure 14.7 a & b
Persistent hyperplastic tunica vasculosa lentis/persistent hyperplastic primary vitreous and persistence of the hyaloid artery in a 7-month-old dog. Note the small lens with a triangular shape and a very thin linear strand, which can be seen extending from the posterior surface of the lens to the optic disc. The pulsating signal obtained on pulsed-wave Doppler examination reveals arterial blood flow in this strand indicating a patent hyaloid artery.

Opacities originating from the posterior segment include vitreous haemorrhage or inflammation. In fresh vitreous bleeding the whole vitreous contains fine moving echoes. When organising, vitreous haemorrhage tends to form clots which appear like larger echogenic patchy zones and/or membranes, which can lead to vitreo-retinal adhesions and secondary tractional retinal tears or detachments. Endophthalmitis also leads to multiple small moving echoes in the whole vitreous and is difficult to differentiate from fresh bleeding. It seems that in uveitis the echoes are less extended and remain nearer to the retina. Synchisis and hyalosis are both degenerative conditions of the vitreous which lead to strong punctual echoes disseminated in the vitreous. When these echoes are seen together with an anechoic zone a few millimetres preretinally, vitreous detachment is likely.

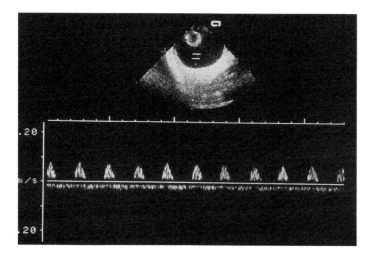

(b)

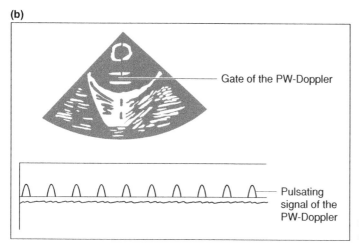

Gate of the PW-Doppler

Pulsating signal of the PW-Doppler

Figure 14.7 a & b
(*continued*)

Subhyaloid (preretinal) haemorrhage usually does not clot. Dispersed mobile echoes are visible in the subhyaloid space.

Ocular trauma

After blunt or sharp ocular trauma, pupillary abnormalities and poor dilation as well as ocular haemorrhage are factors often precluding the opthalmoscopic exam. In these cases, sonography is indicated to assess the integrity of intra-ocular structures and of the globe, and to check for the presence and localisation of a foreign body (Figure 14.8). After an insult, traumatic uveitis or an endophtalmitis can occur. These diseases can lead to fibrin deposition, which, when accumulated in the anterior chamber, can result in

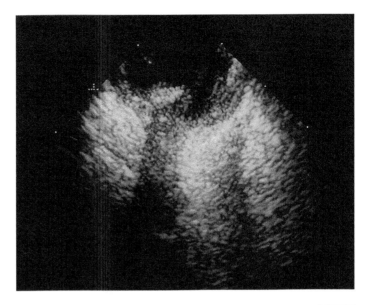

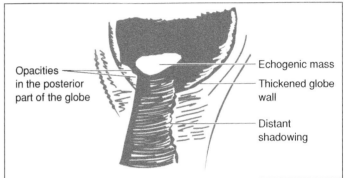

Figure 14.8 Intra-ocular foreign body (piece of glass) and retinal detachment in a 7-year-old collie. An echogenic mass producing distant shadowing is seen in the caudal part of the globe. Note also the irregularly thickened posterior globe wall and the membrane-like opacities in the posterior part of the globe.

secondary glaucoma. Phthisis bulbi is another possible consequence of trauma and is due to a deficiency of the vascularisation of the globe.

Contour of the globe

In glaucoma the globe becomes diffusely enlarged. In cats, the anterior segment appears more enlarged respective to the posterior part of the globe. Sometimes the shape of the globe becomes abnormal and an outpouching can be seen (staphyloma).

Compression of the globe occurs often secondary to an orbital mass. Thickening of the posterior globe wall can be seen in association with posterior scleritis or uveitis (Figure 14.9).

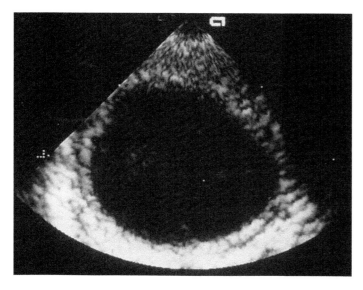

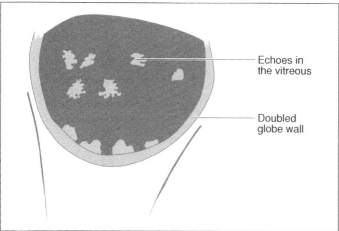

Echoes in
the vitreous

Doubled
globe wall

Figure 14.9 Ocular
globe of a 2-year-old
cat with uveitis
secondary to FIP. Due
to thickening and
oedema, the globe
wall appears doubled.
Some echoes are seen
in the vitreous.

An anechoic space visible between the outer sclera and
the orbital fat is usually due to fluid accumulation in the
Tenon's space. This space is in continuity with the optic
nerve sheath and forms the so-called 'T sign'. This fluid
accumulation is sometimes seen in inflammatory, traumatic
or compressive processes in relation with the optic nerve.

Optic disc

Optic disc cupping is usually seen in association with glaucoma, but can also be detected in normal dogs (Figure 14.10).

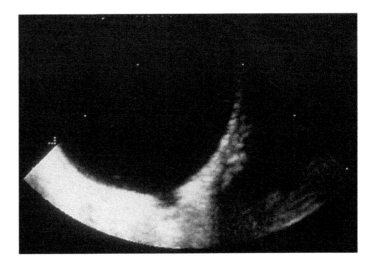

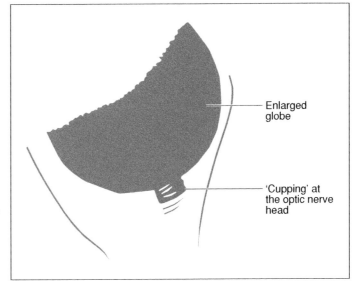

Enlarged globe

'Cupping' at the optic nerve head

Figure 14.10
Enlarged globe and excavation of the globe wall at the optic nerve head (cupping) in a dog with glaucoma and an intra-ocular pressure of 68 mm Hg.

Protruding of the optic disc (papilledema or papillitis) occurs sometimes in neoplastic or inflammatory disease of the optic nerve as well as with an increased intracranial or cerebral spinal pressure (Figure 14.11).

Coloboma of the papilla is a congenital anomaly that belongs to the Collie eye syndrome. Fissures or pits with secondary posterior vitreal herniation around the optic disc can sometimes be seen.

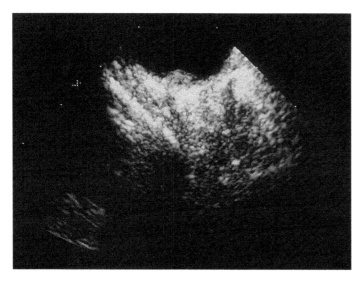

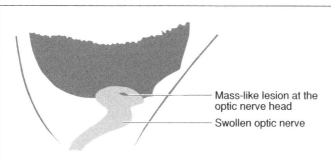

Mass-like lesion at the optic nerve head

Swollen optic nerve

Figure 14.11
Posterior part of the globe in an 8-year-old poodle. There is a small mass-like lesion just at the level of the optic nerve head. The optic nerve itself can be seen as a hypoechoic strand running posteriorly. The papilla of the contralateral eye has the same enlarged appearance. The dog was euthansed because of progressive blindness and a neuropathological exam was performed; histology exam of the brain revealed a granulomatous encephalitis with optic nerve neuritis.

Lens

Subluxation of the lens is difficult to see sonographically but can eventually be assessed using a strict axial scanning plane (Figure 14.12). The appearance of posterior luxation has already been described (see ocular masses).

Orbital sonography

Imaging technique

The retrobulbar area is difficult to evaluate, as conventional radiography is limited to bony diseases or radio-opaque foreign bodies. High quality images of the orbita and peri-orbita can be obtained with CT and MRI but this is costly and general anaesthesia is required. Due to its availability

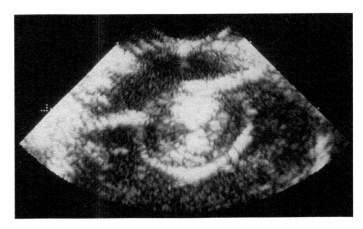

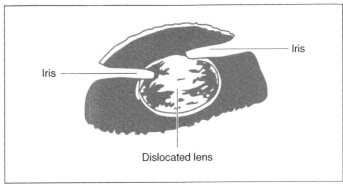

Figure 14.12 Anterior part of the eye in a dog with a subluxated lens. Note the slightly caudally dislocated lens and the asymmetric position of the iris. The lens contains hyperechoic spots due to cataract formation.

and relatively low cost, ultrasound is the imaging technique of choice for the soft tissues of the retrobulbar area in veterinary patients. Ultrasonography is however limited when the lesion extends beyond the boundaries of the bony orbit and peri-orbital or intracranial involvement is suspected.

The orbital space is a conical cavity. This conus is shallower in brachycephalic than in dolichocephalic breeds. In dogs and cats, only the medial wall and parts of the orbital roof are osseous. The orbita is delineated medially by the frontal and palatine bones that form a curved, highly echogenic line with acoustic shadowing. In the orbital floor lie the zygomatic salivary gland, the pterygoid muscles and a fat cushion. Laterally, the broad orbital ligament forms the rostral limit of the orbita whereas the posterior part is made out of the masseter muscle, the zygomatic arch and the vertical mandibular ramus. The frontal sinus lies dorsally, the maxillary sinus and the alveoli of the caudal maxillary teeth lie ventrally to the orbita. The lachrymal gland lies dorsolaterally to the globe. The nasal cavity and ethmoid lie between both medial orbital walls. The orbita is a definite space and alteration in the volume of its contents will shift the position of the globe.

The main indications for sonography of the peri-orbital region include exophthalmos, draining peri-orbital wounds, trauma and suspected foreign body.

There are two main approaches for orbital screening: the transocular approach, which is the same as described for ocular sonography, and the para-ocular (or temporal) approach, which has been described in dogs.

Normal appearance

On sonographic exam, the orbit appears highly reflective due to orbital fat. The other orbital structures appear less echogenic. Among these, the extraocular muscles, the optic nerve, the lachrymal gland and orbital vessels are generally examined during orbital screening.

The extraocular muscles are visible as hypoechoic bands that form a cone, which contains orbital fat and the optic nerve.

The optic nerve is difficult to visualise as such when scanning axially through the optic disc because the disc is highly reflective and causes a V-shaped shadowing. Transocular scanning avoiding the optic nerve head or a temporal scanning allows the examination of the optic nerve, which is a low-reflective elongated structure surrounded by the more echogenic dural sheath.

Except for the largest orbital vessels like the ethmoid artery on the medial orbital wall, ciliary vessels along the caudal globe wall and some orbital veins like the superior and inferior ophthalmic veins, the topographic examination of the orbital vessels necessitates colour or power Doppler. It is probable that vascular malformations such as arterio-venous fistulas or orbital varix are seen as large pulsatile or non-pulsatile anechoic tubular structures but the sonographic appearance of these diseases has not yet been published in veterinary medicine.

Abnormal appearance

Orbital cellulitis

In a patient with exophthalmos with no visible mass lesion, with a highly echogenic and inhomogeneous orbital fat and

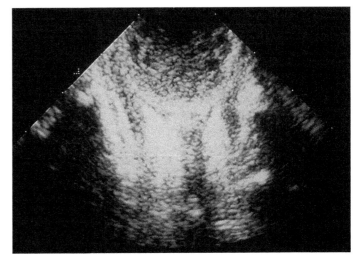

Figure 14.13
Panophthalmitis and orbital cellulitis in a 10-year-old Shih Tzu. Echogenic opacities are filling the posterior part of the globe. The globe wall is thickened. A thin anechoic space is seen behind it and around the proximal part of the optic nerve indicating the presence of fluid in the episcleral space and probably in the optic nerve sheath. The orbital space appears hyper-echogenic, especially between the extra-ocular muscles.

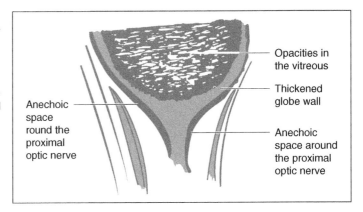

a rounded posterior extremity of the orbital cone, orbital cellulitis must be suspected (Figure 14.13).

Orbital cellulitis is often secondary to diseases of the caudal maxillary teeth or to a penetrating mucosal lesion in the mouth, with or without foreign body. Less frequently, an infectious process from the zygomatic gland, paranasal sinuses or proximal nasolachrymal duct can lead to orbital cellulitis.

Orbital mass lesions

Most of the solid orbital masses can be visualised if they are hypoechoic and relatively well delineated. Among them, lymphoma is often encountered. Osteosarcoma, fibrosarcoma and nasal adenocarcinoma are also commonly diagnosed orbital tumours. Like any mass lesion in the orbit, they often lead to compression of the posterior globe wall. Complex and hyperechoic masses which can be difficult to delineate also occur in the retrobulbar space. Osteogenic tumours of the orbita are often strongly echogenic and arise from the medial or dorsal aspect of the orbita.

Sometimes a mass cannot be assessed in its whole extension. This is the case in masses with poor transmission of the sound waves but also in masses which extend from the peri-orbital area, like nasal adenocarcinomas invading through the medial orbital wall. In such a case the mass but also the interrupted echogenic line of the damaged bone will be seen (Figure 14.14). Metastasis of a malignant melanoma from the eye or from the oral cavity is possible

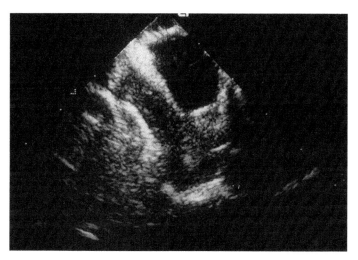

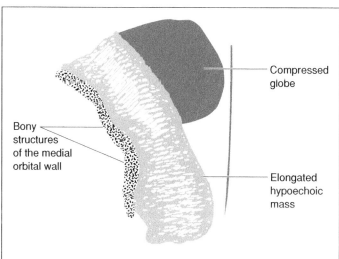

Figure 14.14
Exophthalmos in a 14-year-old cat. An elongated hypoechoic mass compresses the globe medially. The bony structures of the medial orbital wall are interrupted. This mass was a nasal adeno-carcinoma extending into the orbita.

and the extension of a primary intra-ocular melanoma into the orbit through the ocular wall is sometimes observed in spite of the strong sclera barrier.

Benign orbital masses (granulomas, histiocytomas) are infrequent and for this reason cytological or histological examination of every orbital mass is indicated. These diagnostic procedures can be performed under sonographic guidance.

Retrobulbar abscesses have been described in veterinary medicine. They can present as hypo- to anechoic more or less well delineated areas but can also show variable echogenicity patterns and thickened or irregular walls (Figure 14.15). It

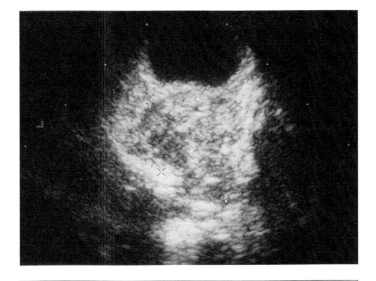

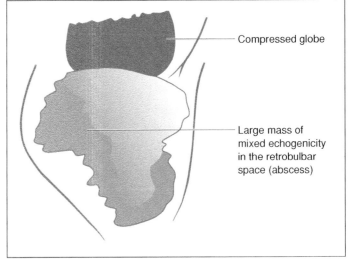

Figure 14.15
Exophthalmos in a 4-year-old cat. A large mass (18 × 21 mm) with a mixed echogenicity is seen in the retrobulbar space, compressing the posterior globe wall. This mass was an abscess.

Compressed globe

Large mass of mixed echogenicity in the retrobulbar space (abscess)

is often not possible to differentiate these from solid masses on the basis of the echographic exam alone.

Cystic lesions in the orbita are almost exclusively zygomatic salivary mucocele or, rarely, lachrymal cysts.

Suggested Reading

Atta, H. R. (1996) *Opthalmic Ultrasound*. Churchill Livingstone, New York.

Boroffka, S. A. E. B., Verbruggen, A. M., Boevé, H. M., *et al.* (1998) Ultrasonographic Diagnosis of Persistent Hyperplastic Tunica Vasculosa Lentis/Persistent Hyperplastic Primary Vitreous in Two Dogs. In: *Veterinary Radiology & Ultrasound*, **39**:4, pp. 440–444.

Boydell, P. (1991) Ultrasonographic Differentiation of Vitreous Membranes and Retinal Detatchment in the Dog. Abstract International Society of Veterinary Ophthalmologists Meeting, Vienna, Austria.

Duncan, D. E. & Peiffer, R. L. (1991) Morphology and Prognostic Indicators of Anterior Uveal Melanomas in Cats. In: *Progress in Veterinary and Comparative Opthalmology*, **1**:1, pp. 25–32.

Dziezyc, J., Hager, D. A. & Millichamp, N. J. (1987) Two-dimensional Real-time Ocular Ultrasonography in the Diagnosis of Ocular Lesions in Dogs. In: *Journal American Animal Hospital Association*, **23**, pp. 501–508.

Gelatt-Nicholson, K. J., Gelatt, K. N., Brooks, D. E., *et al.* (1999) Doppler Imaging of the Ophthalmic Vasculature of the Normal Dog: Blood Velocity Measurements and Reproducibility. In: *Veterinary and Comparative Opthalmology*, **2**, pp. 97–105.

Hansson, K. & Ulhorn, M. (1998) Retrobulbar Foreign Body: Ultrasonographic Diagnosis and Surgical Guidance. Abstract 5th Annual European Association of Veterinary Diagnostic Imaging Conference, Sweden.

Hendrix, D. V. H. & Gelatt, K. N. (2000) Diagnosis, Treatment and Outcome of Orbital Neoplasia in Dogs: A Retrospective Study of 44 Cases. In: *Journal of Small Animal Practice*, **41**, pp. 105–108.

Lieb, W. E. (1993) Color Doppler Sonography of the Eye and Orbit. In: *Current Opinion in Opthalmology*, **4**:3, pp. 68–75.

Mattoon, J. S. & Nyland, T. G. (2002) Eye. In: *Small Animal Diagnostic Ultrasound*, pp. 305–324. W. B. Saunders Co., Philadelphia.

Morgan, R. V. (1989) Ultrasonography of Retrobulbar Diseases in the Dog and Cat. In: *Journal of the American Animal Hospital Association*, **25**, pp. 393–399.

Ramsey, D. T., Gerding, P. A. & Losonsky, J. M. (1994) Comparative Value of Diagnostic Imaging Techniques in a Cat with Exophthalmos. In: *Veterinary and Comparative Opthalmology*, **4**, pp. 198–202.

Rantanen, N. W. & Ewing, R. L. (1981) Principles of Ultrasound Application in Animals. In: *Veterinary Radiology*, **22**, pp. 196–203.

Samsom, J., Barnett, K. C. & Dunn, K. A. (1994) Ocular Disease Associated with Hypertension in 16 Cats. In: *Journal of Small Animal Practice*, **35**, pp. 604–611.

Schiffer, S. P., Rantanen, R. W., Leary, G. A., *et al.* (1982) Biometric Study of the Canine eye, using A-mode Ultrasonography. In: *American Journal of Veterinary Research*, **43**:5, pp. 836–830.

Schmid, V. & Murisier, N. (1996) Color Doppler Imaging of the Orbit in the Dog. In: *Veterinary and Comparative Opthalmology*, **6**, pp. 35–44.

Schoester, S. V., Dubielzig, R. R. & Sullivan, L. (1993) Choroidal Melanoma in a Dog. In: *Journal of the American Veterinary Medical Association*, **203**:1, pp. 89–91.

Stuhr, C. M. & Scagliotti, R. H. (1996) Retrobulbar Ultrasound in the Mesaticephalic and Dolichocephalic Dog using a Temporal Approach. In: *Veterinary and Comparative Opthalmology*, **6**, pp. 91–99.

Chapter 15

Ultrasound of Exotic Species

Sharon Redrobe

In this chapter on ultrasound of exotic species, each group of species is dealt with separately and a list of the indications for ultrasound in that group is given. Ultrasonography has a variety of uses in exotic animal species, e.g. sex determination of monomorphic species, assessment of reproductive status, detection and monitoring of pregnancy, evaluation of abnormal structures and organs and to obtain ultrasound-guided biopsies of specific organs or lesions. The use of ultrasonography in many of these species is limited only by the physical size of the specimen and hence the machine capabilities. Therefore, with appropriate equipment all the procedures detailed in this chapter can be achieved by the interested clinician with a little practice. For the enthusiastic exotic sonographer, a full range of transducers allowing the full range of Doppler ultrasound interrogations and M-mode measurements to be made is necessary.

Mammals

Indications

Indications for ultrasound in exotic mammalian species with a list of potential causes are listed in Table 15.1.

Imaging procedure

In some species such as the chinchilla, ultrasound examination through the fur is possible if sufficient gel is used to exclude air, however some hair removal is required in most species. This should be minimised as large areas of hair loss can predispose the patient to hypothermia. Care should be taken not to wet or chill small mammals excessively, because hypothermia, especially during sedation or general anaesthesia, can be fatal. Similarly, the use of alcohol-based skin preparations should be avoided.

Table 15.1 Conditions for which ultrasonography is a useful diagnostic tool in mammals.

Problem	Species	Possible causes	Ultrasonography
Renal/liver disease	All	Infection Degeneration Toxicity Neoplasia	Examination of organ Ultrasound-guided biopsy

Pregnancy
  toxaemia
	Guinea pigs,
	rabbit
		Large fetus
		Dead fetus
		Obesity
			Pregnancy diagnosis
			Determine whether fetus
			  alive or dead

Diarrhoea	Rabbit	Coccidiosis	Hepatobiliary tree dilation
			  associated with hepatic
			  coccidiosis

Vomiting	Ferret	Ingestion of foreign body Gastritis Lymphoma Gastric neoplasia	Detection of foreign body, gastric wall abnormality
Haematuria	All	Urolithiasis Cystitis Neoplasia bladder Neoplasia uterus Renal infection Normal red pigments	Investigation of urogenital tract

Lameness
Lethargy
Weakness
	Ferret	Insulinoma
		Lymphoma
		Adrenal gland disease
		Anaemia (persistent oestrus)
		Aleutian disease
		Canine distemper
		Cardiomyopathy
			Examination of pancreas,
			  lymph nodes, adrenal
			  glands, heart

Cervical
  lymphadenopathy
	Guinea pig	*Streptococcus zooepidemicus*
		  infection
			Examination of abdominal
			  lymph nodes (not
			  detectable unless
			  enlarged)

Ovarian
  enlargement
	All	Cystic ovaries	Fluid-filled cysts attached
			  to ovary

Uterine
  enlargement
	All	Pyometra
		Uterine adenocarcinoma (rabbit)
		Uterine haemorrhage/
		  ruptured venous aneurysm
			Ultrasonography of uterus
			  to differentiate lesions

Proptosis	Rabbit	Abscess or neoplasia (intra-
		  ocular or retrobulbar)
			Examination of retrobulbar
			  area to differentiate

In general, the anatomy of the small mammal is similar to the more familiar domestic species and therefore positioning of the animal and placement of the transducer is similar. The levels of stress caused by physical restraint and the risk of trauma to the animal and handler must also be taken into account when attempting prolonged physical restraint for ultrasonography. In all but the most tractable individuals, it is often preferable to sedate or perform general anaesthesia. Short acting or reversible agents are preferred and are listed in Appendices 1–6, pp. 330–331.

Ultrasonography of the abdominal organs may be hindered by the presence of a large hindgut in the herbivore species. Ultrasonography of the bladder, uterus, liver and spleen is possible percutaneously via the ventral abdomen in most species. Ultrasonography of the kidneys and ovaries is easier percutaneously via the flank. Rabbits and rodents possess an open inguinal canal and the testes may therefore ascend into the abdomen when palpated. Ultrasonography of these organs is facilitated by general anaesthesia.

Normal appearance

The normal sonographic anatomy of the rabbit is seen in Diagram 15.1.

Monogastric mammals such as murine rodents (rat, mouse, gerbil, hamster) and ferrets possess similar anatomy

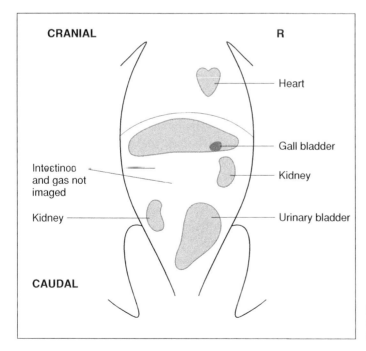

Diagram 15.1 Normal ultrasonographic anatomy of the rabbit.

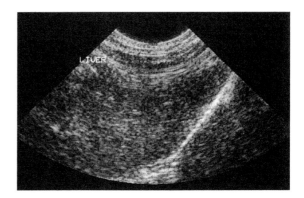

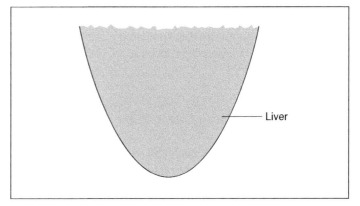

Liver

Figure 15.1
Ultrasound image
of the rabbit liver.

to the more familiar cat or dog. The herbivorous species
such as the rabbit, guinea pig and chinchilla, possess a large
hindgut for microbial digestion which can hinder the ultrasonographic process. The normal rabbit liver is shown in
Figure 15.1.

Heart rates in the small mammals are much faster than
the dog or human (for which most machines are designed).
In the rabbit, heart rate varies between 150 and 250 beats
per minute, whereas the mouse may have a rate of over 250
beats per minute. The ultrasound machine must have a
frame rate or update rate fast enough to image this or the
cardiac image will merely be a blur. Echocardiography has
been described in the rabbit, the mouse and the rat. The
following measurements are considered the most useful and
accurate in small mammals

1 left ventricular systolic time intervals;
2 right ventricular systolic time intervals;
3 right ventricular end-diastolic dimension;

4 left atrial internal dimension;

5 left ventricular end-diastolic and end-systolic dimensions;

6 systolic slope of the interventricular septum;

7 mid-diastolic partial closure of the mitral valve (EF slope); and

8 systolic slope of the posterior aortic wall.

Abnormalities

Hepatic lipidosis is an important sequel to anorexia and is relatively common in rabbits, chinchillas, guinea pigs and ferrets. From the ultrasound scan a homogeneously increased echogenicity is suggestive of this diagnosis. An ultrasound-guided biopsy may be performed to allow histological investigation of liver disease.

Although splenomegaly may be a 'normal' finding in ferrets, abnormalities in the splenic parenchyma detected by ultrasonography indicate pathology.

Ultrasonography has been used to detect urolithiasis in small mammals. Discrete calculi with associated acoustic shadowing may be detected in the urinary bladder and associated bladder wall thickening may also be found. Urethrolithiasis may be detected using ultrasonography but care must be taken to differentiate between calculi in the urethra and the os penis in species such as the guinea pig, chinchilla and ferret where this is present. Renal ultrasonography is frequently performed and infarcts, cysts, abscesses may all be detected. Ultrasonography may be used to perform an ultrasound-guided biopsy of the kidney in order to perform histology and reach a definitive diagnosis. Urethral obstruction in the male ferret may be due to prostatic hyperplasia as a response to adrenal disease. Abdominal ultrasonography will reveal adrenalomegaly in these cases.

Ovarian cysts have been reported in guinea pigs and detected using ultrasonography. Clinical signs include anorexia, alopecia, or depression. Ultrasonographic features of fluid-filled cysts of 2 cm to 3 cm diameter included compartmentalisation and connection to the ovary. Uterine adenocarcinoma and pyometra may be diagnosed and differentiated by ultrasonography in the rabbit.

Subcutaneous and abdominal masses in guinea pigs may be due to cervical adenitis and abdominal lymph node abscessation caused by *Streptococcus zooepidemicus*. Therefore, abdominal ultrasonography should be used to investigate the possibility of abdominal lymph node enlargement when cervical lymph node enlargement is detected on clinical examination.

Ocular disease in small mammals may be investigated using ultrasonography. Intra-ocular abscess and neoplasia have been reported in many small mammals and may be detected using ultrasonography. Exophthalmos may be caused by a retrobulbar mass, e.g. neoplasia or abscess and is commonly seen in pet rabbits. Ultrasonography of the retrobulbar area via the eye is a useful diagnostic aid in such cases.

Sedative or anaesthetic drugs used to restrain small mammalian species may affect myocardial contractility and it is important to be aware of this so that the ultrasound findings can be interpreted correctly. For example, myocardial contractility in rabbits is higher with isoflurane/nitrous oxide anaesthesia than halothane/nitrous oxide anaesthesia. In addition, ultrasonography has been used to evaluate heart damage caused by general anaesthetic agents. An example of this is myocardial fibrosis, which is associated with ketamine/xylazine anesthesia in rabbits and has been detected during echocardiography. Cardiomyopathy is a relatively common post mortem finding in aged rabbits. As longevity of pet rabbits increases, the incidence of heart failure and atherosclerosis also increases. Dilated cardiomyopathy is the most common cardiac abnormality in ferrets. Confirmation is by demonstrating a reduced fractional shortening on ultrasonography. Echocardiography is recommended in rabbits showing dyspnoea or signs of exercise intolerance. A ventricular septal defect has been demonstrated in a rabbit presenting with chronic dyspnoea and it is likely that as this technique becomes more widely used in the small mammal patient, more conditions will be identified *in vivo*.

Reptiles

Common pet reptile species include a variety of lizards, snakes and chelonia (tortoises, terrapins and turtles). These include the Green iguana (*Iguana iguana*), Leopard gecko (*Eublepharis macularius*), Water dragon (*Physignathus cocinus*), Boa constrictor (*Boa constrictor constrictor*), Burmese python (*Python molurus bivittatus*), Royal python (*Python regius*), corn snakes and rat snakes (*Elaphe* spp.), king snakes (*Lampropeltis getulus*), garter snakes (*Thamnophis* spp.), Herman's tortoise (*Testudo hermanni*), Greek/Spur thighed tortoise (*Testudo graeca*), American box turtle (*Terrapene* spp.), and Red-eared terrapin/slider (*Pseudemys scripta elegans*).

Ultrasound is a useful addition to radiography and may prove superior in many cases particularly in chelonia where the bony shell severely limits the diagnostic potential of survey radiographs. Previously, contrast studies have been used to provide more information.

High resolution equipment is required in all but the largest patients. 7.5 MHz/10 MHz sector transducers with a small footprint are recommended. Acoustic coupling gel is applied liberally to the skin and transducer and a stand-off pad is required in patients weighing less than 200 g. Alternatively, the patient is partially submerged in warm water and the transducer placed underwater at an appropriate distance from the animal to achieve the optimum image.

Indications

Conditions where ultrasonography may prove useful in reptiles are described in Table 15.2.

Table 15.2   Conditions for which ultrasonography is a useful diagnostic tool in reptiles.

Problem	Clinical signs	Possible causes	Ultrasonography
Subcutaneous swelling	Subcutaneous swelling	Abscess Trauma Parasitic cyst/worm Neoplasia Granuloma (bacterial, fungal)	Direct imaging of mass to differentiate between parasite (often live and movement seen), abscess (homogenous) and neoplasia (heterogeneous and vessels coon in most cases)
Nutritional osteodystrophy Metabolic bone disease	Pathological fractures Lameness Weakness Fibrous osteodystrophy Muscle tremors Seizures Tetany	Calcium deficiency Improper calcium: phosphorous ratio Lack of vitamin D3 Lack of ultraviolet light Protein deficiency Disease of kidneys, liver, small intestine, thyroid or parathyroid – rare	May see various renal pathologies or may be associated with parathyroid gland enlargement and/or fibrosis
Visceral gout	Lethargy Anorexia Weight loss	Inappropriate diet Dehydration Renal failure	Affected organs reveal hyperechoic areas of uric acid deposition

Table 15.2 (*continued*)

Problem	Clinical signs	Possible causes	Ultrasonography
Vitamin A deficiency	Swollen eyes	Dietary deficiency – meat only	Renal damage Investigate presence of renal gout
Vitamin B1 deficiency	Neurological signs (fitting, twitching)	Dietary deficiency – feeding frozen fish without supplementing with B1	Cardiomyopathy may develop with decreased fractional shortening, and cardiomegaly, especially atrial dilation
Respiratory disease	Nasal discharge Open mouth breathing Extended neck/ head Cyanosis	Poor husbandry Lack of exercise Poor ventilation Incorrect temperature Bacterial/fungal	Thick exudate or fluid-filling lungs can be detected ultrasonographically
Renal disease	Lethargy Constipation	Poor diet Advanced age Dehydration	Investigate size and internal structure of kidneys Investigate presence of gout
Constipation	Swollen coelom Low/no faecal production	Hypocalcaemia Intestinal obstruction due to foreign body Neoplasia Enlarged kidneys Endoparasites	
Dystocia, egg retention	Straining Lethargy Cloacal discharge	Lack of nesting site Oviduct infection Oversized eggs Debilitation	Calcified egg can be imaged Infertile ovum and live fetuses can be differentiated in live-bearing species
Pre-ovulatory follicular stasis	Swollen abdomen Constipation Anorexia	Unknown Lack of nesting site Poor nutritional status Poor husbandry for nesting	Pre-ovulatory follicles readily distinguished from post-ovulatory eggs Coalesced follicular masses detected Coelomic fluid detected
Cloacal prolapse	Part of distal intestinal tract everted	Calculi Parasitism Polyps Infection Diarrhoea Obstruction of the lower intestinal tract	Intussusception identified Internal masses Foreign body
Post-hibernation anorexia (PHA) (chelonia) Anorexia (all reptiles)	Anorexia on emergence from hibernation	Any concurrent disease Frost damage to retina Aural abscess Rhinitis Pneumonia PHA is NOT a diagnosis	Investigation of systemic disease Detection of hepatic lipidosis

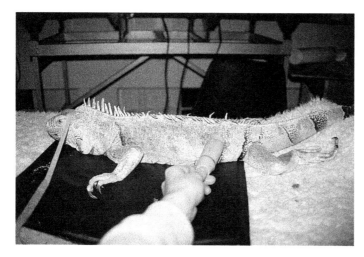

Figure 15.2 Correct positioning of the iguana for lateral flank ultrasonography of gonads.

Imaging procedure

The ribcage in the lizard generally extends more caudally than in mammals, such that in the skink this extends almost to the pelvis. This may cause acoustic shadowing when attempting to scan the caudal coelom. The animal is usually scanned without sedation or anaesthesia but is manually restrained in a vertical position with the head uppermost and the ventral surface facing the ultrasonographer. The lizard may also be scanned through the flank when positioned in dorsal recumbency. This approach is especially useful to rapidly identify the gonads (Figure 15.2). The kidneys are positioned within the pelvis and can be imaged by placing the transducer just cranial to the pelvis and directing caudally. As the heart is located within the pectoral girdle, the transducer is placed at the thoracic inlet and directed caudally. Adequate restraint of the head or, at worst, general anaesthesia is required for this technique. In some species the heart may be imaged directly through the sternum.

The relatively small cross-sectional area of even quite long snakes requires high resolution equipment in all but the largest patients. Although aggressive or highly mobile snakes require sedation or light general anaesthesia, more than 80% of snakes will tolerate a conscious examination, bearing in mind that larger species require more handlers. Some snakes react to the pressure of the probe by closing the ribcage ventrally and again general anaesthesia may be required to prevent this reaction. The snake is scanned across the ventral body wall and although in the larger varieties the ribs may not interfere with the ultrasound image, in smaller species acoustic shadowing will be seen. The heart is located by visualising the heartbeat ventrally in the caudal half of the first third of the length of the snake.

The shell and underlying bony plates of the chelonia restrict the positioning of the transducer to the 'acoustic windows' in the inguinal, pre-femoral, axillary and cervical regions where the transducer may be placed in contact with soft tissue (Figure 15.3). In some species, such as the pancake tortoise, the ultrasound examination may be performed through the greatly reduced shell. The heart muscle may

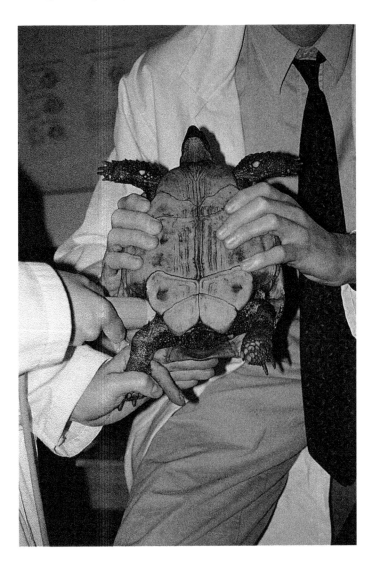

Figure 15.3 Correct positioning of tortoise for ultrasonography.

also be evaluated using M mode, and in patients weighing more than 500 g, Doppler ultrasound may be used to measure stroke volume and identify flow patterns. Common pet chelonia species are usually examined without chemical restraint but aggressive species such as the Red-eared terrapin and Snapper, and species that can close the shell, such as the Box turtle and Hingeback tortoise, require general anaesthesia to prevent injury to the handler and equipment (see Appendix 3, p. 330). If the physical size of the transducer prevents placement between the bony bridge, then an acoustic stand-off is required. Alternatively, the animal and scanner are immersed in a water bath. To access the cervical window, the head and foreleg must be fully extended and pulled to the side. The pre-femoral window is the preferred site for ultrasonographic examination of the caudal coelom. The rear leg is extended to allow placement of the probe on to the soft tissue cranial to the limb. The cervical window is the preferred site to image the heart. The heart is imaged on the midline in the dorsal third of the body. The pre-femoral window is the site preferred to image the liver, gastro-intestinal tract and genito-urinary tract. The bladder is imaged from the pre-femoral window and by angling the transducer towards the midline. The liver is readily imaged through the pre-femoral fossae, and is cranial to the bladder, spanning the midline. Depending on the size of the animal and transducer, the heart may be imaged using the liver as an acoustic window. This does not give as a good an image as when using the cervical window, however.

Normal appearance in the lizard

The relevant anatomy is shown in Diagram 15.2.

The liver is imaged caudal to the elbow. The liver is uniformly echogenic and the anechoic gall bladder is easily seen. The liver is usually less echogenic when compared to the fat pads.

The ovaries may be detected as structures in the mid abdomen, dorsally positioned, containing many small (<0.5 cm) round, hypoechoic areas in the sexually mature female lizard. These areas are pre-vitelline follicles. An ovary containing pre-ovulatory second stage (vitelline) follicles is more easily detected. These large (up to 2.5 cm), round and more hyperechoic structures, are visualised when the

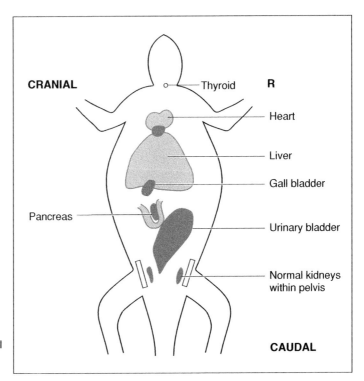

CRANIAL

Thyroid

R

Heart

Liver

Gall bladder

Pancreas

Urinary bladder

Normal kidneys
within pelvis

CAUDAL

Diagram 15.2 Normal ultrasonographic anatomy of the lizard.

transducer is placed almost anywhere on the ventral abdomen from the pelvis to the liver. Once ovulated, the spherical appearance is lost and the structures become ovoid. As the shell is deposited, the oval structure becomes increasingly hyperechoic. The lizard egg appears to have the hypoechoic albumin in the cranial half of the egg and the more hyperechoic yolk is positioned in the ventral half of the egg. The testes are small oval structures in the dorsal abdomen. They are more hyperechoeic than ovaries and have a homogeneous texture, i.e. lack the follicular structure of the ovary.

The thin-walled stomach of the herbivorous lizards is not easily seen with ultrasonography. However, the large intestine can be detected and the large mucosal folds imaged.

The bladder is readily imaged, especially if it is full when it occupies a large portion of the coelom. The anechoic urine may have hyperechoic particles of urates floating within it. The fluid-filled bladder acts as an acoustic window through which to image the other organs.

Large coelomic fat pads are present in well fed lizards. The fat pads have a granular internal structure with hyperechoic septa.

The atrioventricular valves and the hepatic vein leading from the liver to the sinus venosus can be imaged on the longitudinal view of the heart. The atria and ventricles can be imaged and measured. Colour-flow Doppler can be used in animals if the heart is of sufficient size.

Abnormal appearance in the lizard

Enlarged kidneys are more easily imaged than normal ones as they protrude from the pelvic area. Gout in reptiles is usually the deposition of uric acid in soft tissues as a result of dehydration. The hyperechoic deposits may be detected in the kidneys (Figure 15.4).

Abscesses are seen as discrete hyperechoic masses within the liver parenchyma. Hepatic lipidosis is imaged as a diffuse

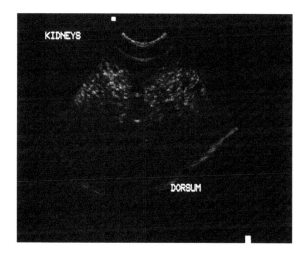

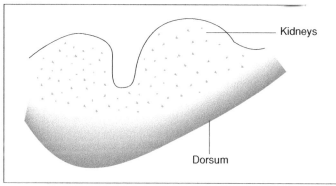

Figure 15.4
Ultrasound image of iguana kidneys. Note the obvious renalomegaly with hyperechoic areas of uric acid deposition (gout).

increase in echogenicity of the liver parenchyma. Pre-ovulatory egg binding in iguanas is a common problem in clinical practice. Radiography of the abdomen will reveal multiple, round, soft tissue masses in the cranial abdomen. The caudal abdomen will show a loss of serosal detail due to fluid accumulation. Ultrasonography is particularly useful in those cases where the ova are small in size and difficult to see on radiography or cannot be differentiated from ovulated eggs on radiography.

Normal appearance in the snake

The relevant anatomy is shown in Diagram 15.3. Note that snakes do not possess a urinary bladder.

The liver is imaged caudal to the heart. This appears as a uniformly moderately hyperechoic organ (similar to the mammalian liver) in the first half of the second third of the snake (Figure 15.5). The fat pads may fill the whole abdominal area of a well fed or obese snake. These appear to be more echogenic than the liver with hyperechoic septa within them. In 'normal' weight snakes the fat pads are often not readily identifiable.

The stomach may be located at the caudal edge of the liver if it contains food particles or fluid. The triad of the

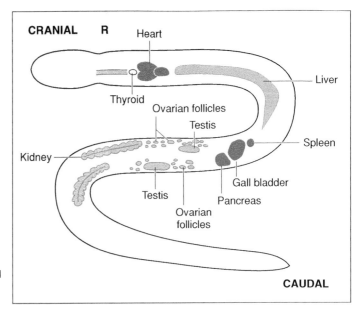

Diagram 15.3 Normal ultrasonographic anatomy of the snake.

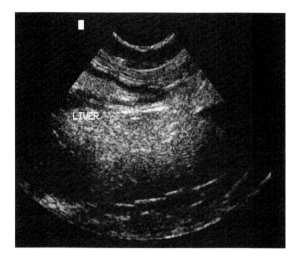

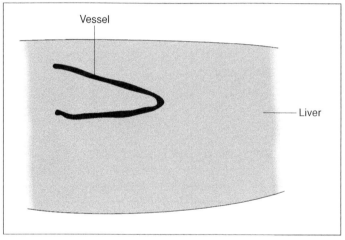

Figure 15.5
Ultrasound image of the normal liver in the snake.

spleen, pancreas and gall bladder serves as a useful landmark in the middle of the snout–vent length of the snake, caudal to the liver yet cranial to the gonads and kidneys. The gall bladder appears as an anechoic focal area (Figure 15.6). The spleen is a small regular sphere, slightly more hyperechoic than the liver and only seen in larger snakes. The pancreas is often indiscernible but may be seen as a less hyperechoic form in the group. The gonad is imaged as oval, hyperechoic structures caudal to the gall bladder/spleen/pancreas triad. The right testis is positioned more cranially than the left one. The testes have a uniform echotexture. In larger snakes the deferent duct may be seen as hyperechoic parallel lines

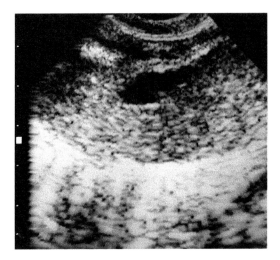

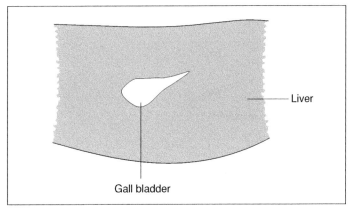

Figure 15.6
Ultrasound image of
the normal gall bladder
in the snake.

originating from the testis. The ovaries are difficult to locate
in the non-cycling female when they may be only the size of
the spleen. In the sexually active, cycling females the ovaries
may fill a large part of the coelom. Follicles on the ovary are
identified as hypoechoic spherical structures. The detection
of the active ovary can be used in the management of breeding colonies such as timing the introduction of the male for
breeding and investigating 'infertility'. Shelled eggs are identified as hyperechoic, dense spherical or oval structures caudal
to the ovaries. The ultrasound may penetrate thin-walled/
leathery eggs. The hypoechoic albumin is often positioned in
one half of the egg with the more echogenic yolk occupying
the other half. The fetus, often moving, can be imaged in
the oviparous snakes and differentiated from infertile egg
masses.

The kidneys are imaged caudal to the gonads. The right kidney is more cranial than the left. They have a similar echotexture to the liver, being uniform throughout. Faecal pellets may be imaged within the large intestine in this area.

Distal to the cloaca, the anal sac is imaged as a hypo- or anechoic round or oval structure. The anal sac is larger in most females compared with males. In males, the inverted hemipenes are located ventral to the anal sac and can be detected as a hyperechoic area on ultrasonography. No equivalent structure is found in females.

With echocardiography the atria, ventricles and atrioventricular valves may be visualised, depending upon the size of the snake. In snakes weighing more than 300 g, the right and left aortic arches may be followed cranially to the common carotid artery. Rib artefact may prove problematic (Figure 15.7).

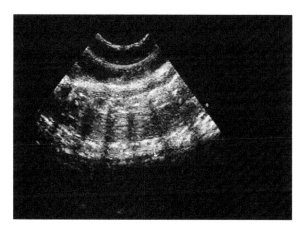

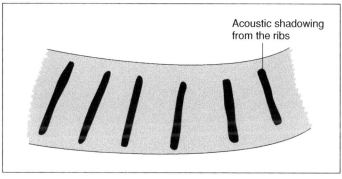

Acoustic shadowing from the ribs

Figure 15.7
Ultrasound image of the snake showing shadowing artefact from ribs.

Abnormal appearance in the snake

Internal masses, or enlargements of the body, are a common presenting sign in snakes and ultrasonography is a useful diagnostic tool in investigating the nature of these lesions. Although the gastro-intestinal tract is not readily identified using ultrasonography, masses within the body of the snake can be identified as arising from the tubular gastro-intestinal tract or other, more solid, organs. The transducer is placed cranial to the mass and moved caudally. The next organ is located (whether kidney, liver, etc.) and it is usually possible to appreciate whether the mass arises from the solid organ or from the dorsal gastro-intestinal tract. In cases of anorexia, the gall bladder is often noted to be greatly enlarged and to fill approximately one third of the diameter of the snake in that area. Abscesses of the anal sac appear hyperechoic.

Normal ultrasonographic anatomy of chelonia

The relevant anatomy is shown in Diagram 15.4.

The liver has a uniformly homogeneous echotexture, similar to mammals (Figure 15.8). The gall bladder can be seen

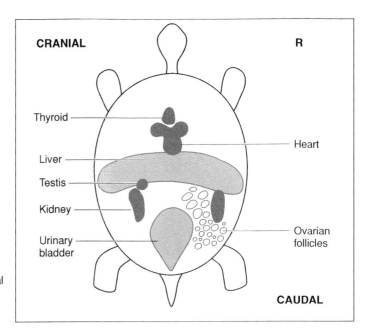

Diagram 15.4 Normal ultrasonographic anatomy of the tortoise.

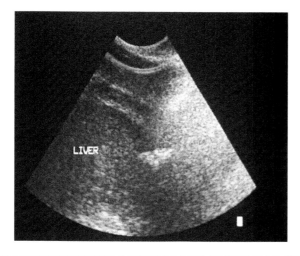

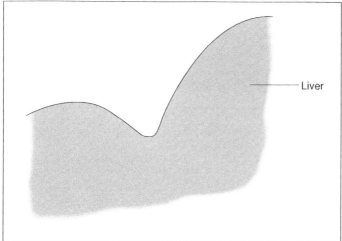

Figure 15.8
Ultrasound image
of the normal liver
in the tortoise.

on the right side as an anechoic structure. The urine-filled
bladder is seen as an anechoic oval structure. Urates may
be detected as hyperechoic specks floating within it.

The ovaries are paired, elongated organs attached to the
peritoneum on either side of the dorsal midline, anterior to
the pelvic girdle. The follicles are more easily imaged against
the background of a large, fluid-filled bladder. When ovulated, the hyperechoic yolk is seen centrally surrounded by
the dark hypoechoic albumin (Figure 15.9). As the shell is
deposited, the dense white hyperechoic margin of yolk
is seen surrounded by the dense fibrous layers of eggshell
increasing the echogenicity of the egg. Ultrasound has been

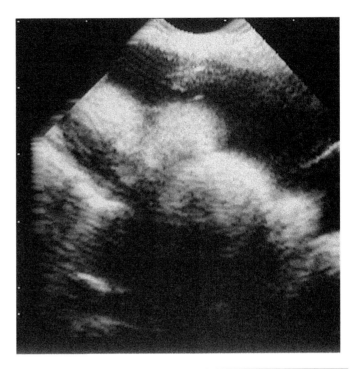

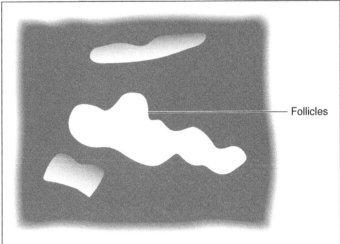

Follicles

Figure 15.9
Ultrasound image of
follicles in the tortoise.

used to detect, count and measure the ovarian follicles and
the oviductal eggs. These numbers can be compared with
the eventual number of eggs laid in the evaluation of dystocia
and the investigation of gestation times. The accurate esti-
mation of the number of follicles or eggs is not possible in

those species that mature large numbers of follicles. Eggs that are in the distal tract may be imaged through the inguinal fossa.

The testes are located cranial and ventral to the kidneys. They appear uniformly echogenic and slightly more hypo-echoic when compared with the adjacent kidneys in chelonia.

Echocardiography has proved rewarding in chelonia. The ventricular and atrial walls, atrioventricular valves and main coronary vessels can be imaged in specimens e.g. Greek (*Testudo graeca*) and Herman's (*Testudo hermanni*) tortoises weighing over 500 g. The blood flow patterns and velocities can be measured using colour Doppler flow and spectral ultrasound.

Abnormal ultrasonographic anatomy of chelonia

Liver abscesses and scarring are detected as a change in the homogeneity of the image. Liver abscesses are commonly reported at post mortem in aged chelonia. These lesions are readily detected using ultrasound when they appear as discrete disruptions to the architecture of the liver. Distinction between abscess and neoplasia does, however, require histopathology. Severe hepatic lipidosis carries a grave prognosis and is seen as a diffuse increase in echogenicity. The finding and extent of hepatic lipidosis in the anorexic chelonian may serve as a prognostic indicator.

Uroliths are imaged as hyperechoic structures within the bladder. The bladder wall is usually only detected in cases of bladder wall thickening caused by such chronic irritation.

Gout in reptiles is usually the deposition of uric acid in soft tissues as a result of dehydration. The hyperechoic deposits may be detected in the kidneys and heart and are a poor prognostic finding.

Ultrasound can penetrate thin-walled eggs of some species, e.g. Red-eared terrapins, to detect the inspissated contents within retained eggs. This has proved a useful guide in determining the age of the egg and hence in diagnosing dystocia.

Abscesses can be detected in the major vessels and associated with the valve leaflets. The relative thickness of the myocardium allows investigation by M-mode ultrasonography in medium-sized patients. Pericardial effusion may occur but must be differentiated from the normal heart chambers. Gross lesions such as major valvular incompetence can be noted.

Birds

Indications

The air sacs within the coelom of bird species severely restrict the use of ultrasonography in these animals. Ultrasonography is therefore most useful in the investigation of the swollen coelom and to allow differentiation between fluid, soft tissue masses and organomegaly. Conditions for which ultrasound may be useful and possible causes for these are given in Table 15.3 below.

Imaging procedure

Tame parrots, trained raptors and other tractable individuals may be examined using physical or minimal chemical restraint. In most cases, it is less stressful to the bird and operator if the bird is lightly anaesthetised using isoflurane (see Appendix 4, p. 331). Feathers interfere with the transmission of the ultrasound beam and must be removed from the area of interest. A minimal area should be plucked as in most species feathers are replaced only once or twice per year. Feathers should be plucked rather than cut as plucking may encourage earlier regrowth. In some species, a featherless tract occurs over the caudal coelom and no plucking is required. Gel is applied to the skin in the normal manner. A 7.5–10 MHz probe with a footprint of less than 2 cm is required to perform ultrasound examinations on most pet parrot, pigeon and raptors species. In most pet birds, weighing between 50 g and 2 kg, the heart rate will exceed 150 beats per minute. The heart itself measures between 0.5 and 2 cm. The ultrasound equipment must therefore have sufficient image definition and adequate frame rate to image the heart effectively.

Transcloacal and transintestinal ultrasonography using high resolution miniaturised probes have been developed in order to circumvent the problems associated with transcoelomic ultrasonography in birds. Transintestinal ultrasonography allows visualisation of the gonads and genital tract, whereas transcloacal ultrasonography is limited to the caudal genital tract. In the normal bird, scanning percutaneously over the coelomic wall, aiming cranially, may contact the liver and allow examination of this organ.

Table 15.3 Conditions for which ultrasonography is a useful diagnostic tool in birds.

Problem	Clinical signs	Possible causes	Ultrasonography
Subcutaneous swelling	Subcutaneous swelling	Abscesses Trauma Neoplasia Granuloma (bacterial, fungal)	Direct imaging of mass to differentiate between abscess (homogenous) and neoplasia (heterogeneous with vessels seen in most cases)
Visceral gout	Lethargy Anorexia Weight loss	Dietary deficiency Dehydration Renal failure	Ultrasonography of affected organs reveal hyperechoic area of uric acid deposition
Vitamin A deficiency	Swollen eyes Swollen peri-ocular sinuses Dehydration	Dietary deficiency, such as sunflower seed diets for parrot	Renal changes Investigate presence of renal gout
Hepatomegaly	Abdominal enlargement Distension Yellow urates	Granuloma Neoplasia Lipidosis Multiple abscesses	Differentiate between homogenous and heterogeneous structure Discrete masses within parenchyma Biliary tree abnormalities
Renal disease	Lethargy Constipation Dehydration Lameness	Poor diet Advanced age Dehydration	Investigate size and internal structure of kidneys Gout
Dystocia Egg retention	Straining Lethargy Cloacal discharge	Lack of nesting site Oviduct infection Oversized eggs Debilitation	Calcified egg
Cloacal prolapse	Part of distal intestinal tract everted	Calculi Parasitism Polyps Infection Diarrhoea Obstruction of the lower intestinal tract	Intussusception Internal masses Foreign body

Normal ultrasonographic anatomy

The relevant anatomy is shown in Diagram 15.5.

Ultrasonography of the liver is facilitated by hepatomegaly. The gall bladder is absent in some species such as the pigeon. The ovaries are not readily imaged unless follicles, an abscess or granuloma enlarge the organ or coelomic fluid is present. The bursa of Fabricius may be identified in juvenile birds. Birds do not possess a urinary bladder.

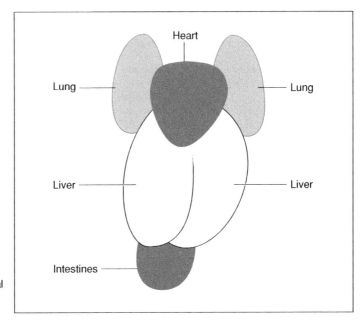

Diagram 15.5 Normal ultrasonographic anatomy of the bird.

Birds do not possess a diaphragm, and so the apex of the heart contacts the cranial edge of the liver directly. The heart may therefore be imaged ultrasonographically by directing the beam through the liver caudad to craniad.

Abnormal ultrasonographically anatomy

Coelomic ultrasonography is enhanced when coelomic fluid is present as this fluid displaces the air-filled air sacs within the coelom. Care should be taken when examining such patients, as they will therefore have a degree of respiratory embarrassment.

Hepatomegaly is a relatively common clinical sign in diseased birds. Ultrasonography may be used to detect masses within the liver parenchyma such as multiple discrete abscesses associated with yersiniosis, or biliary tree neoplasia seen in parrots from the Amazon.

The surrounding air-filled sacs often obscure ultrasonographic imaging of the normal, quiescent ovary, but enlargement of the ovary caused by normal folliculogenesis, or abnormal neoplasia or granuloma often facilitates imaging using ultrasonography. Laminated and thin-shelled eggs can be differentiated from abdominal masses, salpingitis and cystic degeneration using ultrasonography.

Table 15.4 Conditions for which ultrasonography is a useful diagnostic tool in amphibia.

Problem	Clinical signs	Possible causes	Ultrasonographic examination

Bloat	Swollen body	Gastric fermentation
		Air swallowing
		Peritoneal effusions
		  (infection, neoplasia)
			Investigation of presence of
			  fluid, masses, cysts, organ
			  pathology

Cloacal
  prolapse
	Organ protruding
	  from vent
		Foreign body
		Parasites
		Masses
		Gastro-enteritis
			Detection of foreign body
			Parasites
			Masses

Masses	Masses in skin or
	  internal organs
		Parasites
		Bacteria
		Mycobacterium
		Neoplasia
		Spontaneous tumours
		  caused by Lucke
		  tumour herpes virus
			Differentiation of masses

Amphibia

Common pet species include salamanders, firebellied toads, newts and tree frogs.

Indications

Conditions for which ultrasound may be considered useful in these species are listed in Table 15.4.

Imaging procedures

Most amphibians are not accustomed to physical restraint. The delicate skin is easily damaged. It is often therefore preferable to examine these animals using mild sedation/light anaesthesia (see Appendix 5, p. 331). The skin is very absorptive. Although proprietary ultrasound gels are labelled as non-toxic, it is preferable to examine these animals in a water bath rather than risk adverse effects from systemic gel absorption.

Normal ultrasonographic anatomy

The relevant anatomy is shown in Diagrams 15.6 a and 15.6 b.

There is a relatively large amount of body fluid in amphibians, which should not be confused with ascites. In view of

(a) Female frog

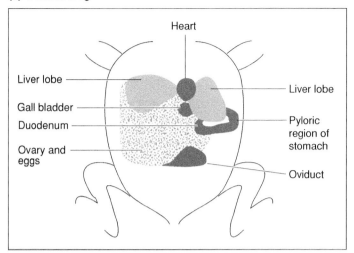

(b) Male frog

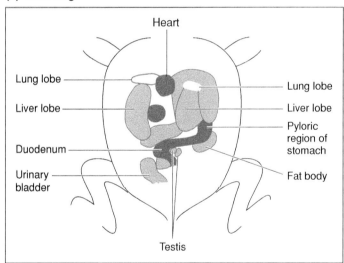

Diagram 15.6 Normal ultrasonographic anatomy of the male and female frog.

the scarce publications on this subject, it is often useful to perform ultrasonography on another individual of the same species in order to establish what is normal or abnormal for that species; many owners will have more than one individual.

Abnormal ultrasonographic anatomy

Bloat is a relatively common presenting sign in amphibia. This may be due to fluid, gas or soft tissue enlargements within the body cavity. Ultrasonography can be used to detect the presence of ascites or organomegaly. Cystic or soft tissue enlargement of organs can be differentiated using ultrasonography.

Cloacal prolapse may occur as a result of ingestion of a foreign body or over large food item, gastro-intestinal tract parasitism or masses of the gastro-intestinal tract (neoplasia, granuloma). Percutaneous ultrasonography may be used to investigate the contents of the gastro-intestinal tract and thus the cause of the prolapse.

Masses of the skin or viscera may arise due to formation of granuloma, neoplasia and parasites. Ultrasonography of the masses may enable differentiation between the types of masses and which organ is affected. Further, a percutaneous biopsy of the mass may be obtained by ultrasound-guided biopsy.

Fish

Common pet species include goldfish and catfish. Larger species, e.g. koi carp, sharks, may be maintained in captivity.

Indications

Conditions for which ultrasound may prove useful in fish are listed below in Table 15.5 along with some potential causes for these.

Table 15.5 Conditions for which ultrasonography is a useful diagnostic tool in fish.

Problem	Clinical signs	Possible causes	Ultrasonography
Corneal opacity	Eye appears cloudy	Trauma Gas bubble trauma Poor water quality Nutritional imbalance Eye fluke	Ocular ultrasonography
Exophthalmia	Enlarged eye	Spring viraemia of carp Swim bladder inflammation Systemic infection	Differentiate intra-ocular from extra-ocular aetiology
Vertebral deformity	Deviation in spine Fish swimming in circles	Nutritional deficiency, e.g. phosphorus, vitamin C Trauma Intramuscular cysts Neoplasia	Examination of spine and surrounding structures

Imaging procedures

Ultrasonography of most fish requires the use of general anaesthesia (see Appendix 6, p. 331). Larger fish such as sharks, may be manually restrained in the water for ultrasonography.

Normal ultrasonographic anatomy

The relevant anatomy is shown in Diagram 15.7.

The skin of many fish is covered with scales, some of which are made of bone and will therefore obstruct the passage of ultrasound. Fish do not possess lungs but have paired sets of gills at the caudal edge of the head. There are two coelomic cavities; the cranial pericardial cavity contains the heart. The caudal peritoneal cavity contains the other viscera and occupies the ventral half of the body, tapering to the anus. The liver lies in the cranial area of the peritoneal cavity, with the majority of the organ on the left side. The gall bladder is on the right side. The spleen may be divided into several parts and is situated on the caudal edge of the stomach. The gastro-intestinal tract is generally divided into stomach, intestine and rectum regions.

There is no urinary bladder but the urine is deposited into a urogenital sinus before exiting via the urogenital orifice. The gas bladder, or swim bladder, is a gas-filled diverticulum

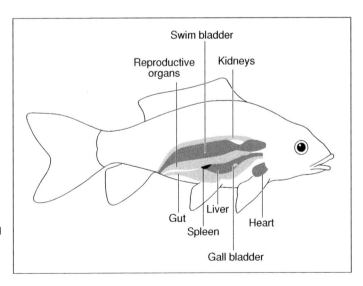

Diagram 15.7 Normal ultrasonographic anatomy of the koi carp.

of the dorsal oesophagus. It occupies the dorsal half of the peritoneal cavity and usually occupies the whole length of this cavity.

Abnormal ultrasonographic anatomy

Vertebral deformities occur in captive fish including sharks. Suggested aetiologies include trauma, nutritional deficiencies, neoplasia and intramuscular cysts. As the spine of many fish, including sharks, is cartilaginous, ultrasonography may be used to image the spinal column and investigate the deformity. Neoplastic or inflammatory changes to the spine are often manifest as proliferative masses of the spine that can be imaged with ultrasonography. Damage or masses within the musculature can be detected using ultrasonography and therefore differentiated from spinal damage.

Corneal opacity may occur as a result of external trauma, poor water quality, nutritional imbalances or parasitic infection of the eye. Ultrasonography may be used to investigate the presence of a parasite within the eye. Exophthalmia may occur due to an intra-ocular problem or as a manifestation of a systemic disease. Ultrasonography of the eye and coelom may assist in the differentiation between the two aetiologies.

Suggested reading

Du Boulay, G. H. & Wilson, O. L. (1988) Diagnosis of Pregnancy and Disease by Ultrasound in Exotic Species. Symposium of the Zoological Society, London, **60**, pp. 135–150.

Hildebrandt, T. B. & Goritz, F. (1999) The Use of Ultrasonography in Zoo Animals. In: *Zoo and Wild Animal Medicine: Current Therapy*, 4th edn, (eds M. E. Fowler & R. E. Millar), pp. 41–54. W. B. Saunders Co., Philadelphia.

O'Grady, J. P., Yeager, C. H. & Thomas, W. (1978) Practical Applications of Real-time Ultrasound Scanning to Problems of Zoo Veterinary Medicine. In: *Journal of Zoo Animal Medicine*, **9**, pp. 52–56.

Pennick, D. G., Stewart, J. S., Paul-Murphy, J., *et al.* (1991) Ultrasonography of the Californian Desert Tortoise (*Xerobates agassizi*): Anatomy and Application. In: *Veterinary Radiography*, **32**:3, pp. 112–116.

Redrobe, S. (1997) Aspects of Ultrasonography of Chelonia. Proceedings of the Association of Reptile and Amphibian Veterinarians, pp. 127–130.

Redrobe, S. (1997) Aspects of Ultrasonography of Lizard. Proceedings of the Association of Reptile and Amphibian Veterinarians, pp. 179–182.

Redrobe, S. (1997) Aspects of Ultrasonography of Snake. Proceedings of the Association of Reptile and Amphibian Veterinarians, pp. 183–186.

Stoskopf, M. K. (1989) Clinical Imaging in Zoological Medicine: A Review. In: *Journal of Zoo Wildlife Medicine*, **20**:4, pp. 396–412.

Appendix

Appendix 1 Agents for sedation and general anaesthesia in mammals.

Drug	Mouse	Rat	Guinea pig	Rabbit	Duration of anaesthesia
Isoflurane	2%	2%	2%	2% (sedate with Hypnorm first)	Maintenance
Hypnorm (Fentanyl/ Fluanisone)	0.2–0.5 ml i/m 0.3–0.6 i/p	As mouse	0.5–1.0 ml/kg i/m	0.2–0.4 ml i/m	30–45 minutes
Hypnorm (Fentanyl/ Fluanisone)/ Diazepam	0.4 ml/kg 5 i/p	0.3 ml/kg 2.5 i/p	1 ml/kg 2.5 i/m	0.3 ml/kg i/m 2 i/p	45–60 minutes
Hypnorm/ Midazolam*	10 ml/kg* i/p	2.7 ml/kg* i/p	8 ml/kg* i/p	0.3 ml/kg i/m 0.5–1 i/v	45–60 minutes
Ketamine/ Medetomidine	200 mg/kg 0.5 i/p	90 mg/kg 0.5 i/p	40 mg/kg i/m 0.5 i/m	35 mg/kg i/m 0.5 i/m	20–30 minutes
Propofol	26 mg/kg i/v	10 mg/kg i/v	–	10 mg/kg i/v	5 minutes

*one part Hypnorm, one part midazolam, two parts water

Appendix 2 Reversal agents for sedative/general anaesthesia agents.

Agent	To reverse	Dose mg/kg	Route
Atipamazole	Any combination using Medetomidine	1	i/m i/p s/c i/v
Buprenorphine	Any combination using Hypnorm	0.05 rabbit; 0.1 small rodents	i/m i/p s/c i/v
Butorphanol	Any combination using Hypnorm	0.3 rabbit; 1 small rodents	i/m i/p s/c i/v

Appendix 3 Anaesthetic agents for reptiles.

Drug	Dosage (mg/kg)	Site
Alphaxalone/alphadolone	6–9	i/v
	9–15	i/m
Ketamine	20–100 (larger dose to smaller animals)	i/m i/p
Propofol	Tortoises 14	i/v
	Lizards 10	
	Snakes 10	
Isoflurane	2–6%	Inhalation

Appendix 4 Anaesthetic agents for use in birds.

Anaesthetic	Dosage (mg/kg)	Comments
Isoflurane	Induction 4%, maintenance 2%, O_2 flow 1–2 litres/minute	Swiftly induces easily handled birds, rapid recovery. 50% N_2O reduces isoflurane dose required
Halothane	Induction 1%, increase to 3%, maintain at 1.5–3%	Cardiac failure if too rapid induction
Ketamine + Diazepam or Midazolam	25 K; 2.5 D i/m	20–30 minutes deep sedation
Ketamine/Medetomidine	Raptors 3–5 K/50–100 M i/m Psittacines 3–7 K/75–150 M i/m	
Propofol	3–5 i/v	Wears off very quickly, care with transfer to gaseous anaesthetic

Appendix 5 Anaesthetic agents for use in amphibia.

Anaesthetic	Tadpoles Newts	Frogs Salamanders	Toads	Comments
Methanesulphate (MS222)	200–500 mg/l	500–2000 mg/l	1–3g/l	To effect, begin with low concentration
Ethyl-4-aminobenzoate (benzocaine)	50 mg/l	200–300 mg/l	200–300 mg/l	Must be dissolved in methanol then added to water as not very soluble. Stock solution may be kept in dark bottle for up to three months
Ketamine	50–150 mg/kg			
Isoflurane, halothane	4–5% bubbled through water			Animals may be intubated using small tubing and placed on moistened towels
Dopram hydrochloride	Empirical dosage			Useful to stimulate breathing

Appendix 6 Anaesthetic agents for use in fish.

Anaesthetic	Dosage (mg/Kg)	Comments
Methanesulphate (MS222)	100 mg/ml	Only licensed product in UK
Ethyl-4-aminobenzoate (benzocaine)	40 g into 1 litre methanol; 11 ml of *this* solution into 9 litres water	Must be dissolved in methanol then added to water as not very soluble. Stock solution may be kept in dark bottle for up to three months

Glossary

A mode	Amplitude mode ultrasound – now largely outdated
Anechoic	Lacking in echoes, so image seen as a black structure on the display
Annular array	A crystal arrangement where the crystal elements are arranged as a bull's eye/target. Found in some mechanical sector transducers
Attenuation	Reduction in intensity of the ultrasound beam as it passes through tissue
Axial resolution	The ability to be able to differentiate two points along the axis of the ultrasound beam – can only be equal to the pulse length of the ultrasound being used
B mode	Brightness mode – most commonly used mode in diagnostic ultrasonography
Comet-tail artefact	Echoes resulting from reverberation within a metallic object
Echogenic	Results in return of echoes and so is usually quite white on the screen
Frame rate	The frequency with which the ultrasound image displayed is replaced
Frequency	The number of cycles per second of the ultrasound wave
Gain	Amplification of returning echoes
Hertz	Unit for frequency, equal to one cycle per second and abbreviated as Hz
Hyperechoic	Brightly reflective, resulting in a bright image
Hypoechoic	Poorly reflective, resulting in a dark image
Isoechoic	Having the same echogenicity as the surrounding medium

Lateral resolution	The ability to differentiate between two structures lying side by side in the path of the ultrasound beam
M mode	Motion mode – a method of measuring thickness and depth and how this changes with time – used especially in cardiac scanning
Phased array	In an arrayed transducer assembly that has very thin rectangular elements arranged side by side. It relies upon electronic beam steering to sweep sound beams over a sector-shaped scanned region. Beam steering is done using electronic time delay in the transmitting and receiving circuits. Used especially for cardiac imaging
Piezoelectric	Pressure electric – these are materials which have the ability to produce acoustic energy in response to electrical energy and vice versa
Rayleigh scatter	A type of scatter of ultrasound waves where the scattering material is much smaller than the wavelength of the incident sound – the most commonly quoted example is that of red blood cells
Reflection	The returning ultrasound waves where they are incident on an interface between tissues of differing acoustic impedance
Refraction	A change in direction of the ultrasound beam as it passes between different tissues, through each of which the ultrasound passes at a different speed
Ring-down artefact	Echo pattern caused by reverberation in a bubble or soft-tissue structure

Index

Printed and bound by CPI Group (UK) Ltd, Croydon, CR0 4YY

Printed and bound by CPI Group (UK) Ltd, Croydon, CR0 4YY

27/10/2024

14580387-0003